Beyond Your Body

The material contained in this book is not intended as medical advice. If you have a medical issued or illness, consult a qualified physician.

Copyright © 2010 by Dr. Gaile Sprissler
All rights reserved. No part of this book may be reproduced or transmitted in any form or by any means, electronic or mechanical, including photocopying, recording, or by any information storage and retrieval system, without permission in writing from the author or publisher.

This edition of the work is protected against unauthorized copying under Title 17, United States Code.

Printed in the United States of America

ISBN 13: 978-1502830746

Beyond Your Body

Pathways To Healing Chronic Pain Conditions

Gaile Sprissler, PhD

CONTENTS

Acknowledgements	vii
Forward	xi
Prologue	xvii
Introduction	
Cause/Cure for Chronic Pain	xxvi
Chapter One	
Chronic Conditions/Quality of Life	1
Chapter Two	
Intra-personal Communication:	7
Chapter Three	
Examining Methods & Procedures:	
Focusing	14
Psychoneuroimmunology	19
Neurolinguistic Programming	29
Placebo response	38
Chapter Four	
Fibromyalgia:	
Symptoms and Beliefs Systems	53
Chapter Five	
What is the Pain Experience?	74
Methods	79
Patterns	79
Commonalities	81
Analysis of Participants	82
Chapter Six	
Discussion and Interpretation	90
Chapter Seven	
Introducing the Ladies	114
Chapter Eight	
Journeying on the Wellness Path	166
Chapter Nine	
Further Exploration	180
Treatment Considerations	187
References	188

ACKNOWLEDGEMENTS

This book is dedicated to the praiseworthy people who inspired me in the conception and completion of this book.

To Dawn Surya, who was a fountain of knowledge; as a scholar, nurse and fibromyalgia patient. She is my spirit sister. Through her prayers, eagerness to instruct, and discuss with me, I learned and sought further information.

To Jean Carney, who propelled me down this path, and convinced me that I would not be satisfied or complete until I did. She helped me articulate my ideas, shared her experiences, and convinced me of the transformation I would experience by pursuing my vision.

To Cindy Wohlford, who paddled my canoe. She encouraged me to persist through any hurdles that are placed in front of me.

To my friends, Jeanine Gerard, Bern Moss and Evelyn Cullet for their help and critiques, and for supporting my work and recognizing the value of this knowledge.

To my contemporaries at the Oak Lawn Writers Group who bore witness to the development, gladly critiqued my endeavors, and provided valuable input as this book was being created.

Many thoughts, ideas, and works contributed to this book. Many mentors, professors, and friends influenced this work. Included also are the many fibromyalgia patients that I have served. They are out there floundering, in search of answers and relief. I pray for all of you and hope alleviation comes soon.

Special thanks to the women who consented to tell me of their experiences and let me into the privacy of their life with fibromyalgia. You are a brave, resourceful and determined group, and I am in awe and proud of all of you.

"I am responsible for the creation of my health. I therefore participated, at some level, in the creation of this illness. I can participate in the healing of this illness by healing myself, which means simultaneously healing my emotional, psychological, physical, and spiritual being."

*-The Energy Medicine Credo,
as quoted by Marcia Emery*

Beyond Your Body

"Inspiration for a healing journey . . .
You are wiser than you know, more courageous than you guess.
You are stronger than you feel in the greatness of your soul."

— *Margery Johnson*

Forward

    During my adult life, I went to the kitchen, not the doctor, when I was not well, and made an herbal tea, took some vitamins, and ate particular foods to heal myself again. I have visited doctors very few times in my life. I have always been very healthy, and tests results have always been normal. I am usually an upbeat, positive person.

    Optimal health is a state where all aspects of the self-care in perfect balance. As a Neuromuscular Therapist, I have a commitment to client education; to help clients care for themselves, as well as to give effective therapy for chronic muscle conditions. I believe that: "Awareness leads to wellness, and my intention is to assist and support my clients on their journey to inner peace and optimal health. This is a path to the body/mind connection of holistic health that includes spiritual, mental, physical and emotional well-being to achieve balance and harmony for the self."

    My profession and passion is to ease and/or relieve chronic pain. This often begins with injury or illness stressing the body, and this causes tension which develops into a complex cycle that drains energy and emotions. The body releases chemicals that stimulate the nerves to send neural messages to the brain. Muscles contract around the painful area and can become habitually contracted, sometimes pressing on nerves, causing more pain; and reducing circulation allowing waste products to accumulate leaving behind a feeling of tiredness and soreness. Over time, poor circulation forms trigger points referring pain elsewhere in the body. Those muscles tense, and the pain cycle spreads. Simple actions become difficult and tiring, and often sleep is interrupted.

While in a Massage Therapy session, the client becomes aware of tension, and how it feels to relax. Varied techniques are used to stimulate the nervous system and send new neural messages to the brain. Also, to stretch and release contracted muscles as well as their trigger points, which increases circulation and waste products are flushed. It also acts on the nervous system to counteract the body's response to stress and pain and optimally, normal movement is restored. Thus, there is renewed energy, relief from chronic pain, and the return to relaxation and restful sleep.

This does not all occur in one session, the results depending on the degree that the client is willing to let go of whatever they are holding, emotional or physically, in a particular area(s). However, often there are other problems in the client's life, and sometimes the old baggage that they have been carrying around. I felt that I needed more information and tools to work with them more effectively. My concern was especially for those clients with chronic conditions, depressed with the duration of their condition, and lacking stimulus to explore research possibilities for themselves. It became important for me to do more research, and develop further additional skills to facilitate their self-healing techniques.

When I entered university as a returning adult student, I also began classes at the Wellness and Massage Institute (WMTI) to become a Massage Therapist. I was beginning to formulate a plan to integrate all of my prior learning and current interests. I decided to obtain an MA in Communications, to teach seminars and workshops on Holistic Health Issues, along with practicing my Massage Therapy. Further, I intended to become a motivational speaker.

During this time, there was a very interesting crossover of information and application between my Communication and Psychology studies at the university, and my chosen elective courses such as stress management, contemporary health issues, transactional analysis, personal and interpersonal growth, nutrition, and ayurvedic healing.

At WMTI, along with the Anatomy, Physiology and Kinesiology classes, I took classes in Wellness Issues and Boundary Issues. I was fascinated by the Wellness Issue courses that opened up Holistic Health implications for our clients and for ourselves. These classes incorporated the exploration of the self, and discussed the emotional, psychological and attitudinal issues the client may be bringing into a session along with their physical problems. I was very interested in learning how to master the ability to help people who are in chronic pain, in a natural way. My many years of interests in vitamins, herbs, and using natural healing techniques seemed to be a natural complement to this program of study.

While pursuing my Masters degree, I conducted a *Lifestyle Change Survey* of 75 people. (Sprissler, 1999) The purpose was to explore an adult's interest in making lifestyle changes for better spiritual, mental, emotional or physical health. The implications of the survey indicate that men were most likely to make lifestyle changes cautiously, and were limited in their expectations of the results. It indicated that women were most likely to make lifestyle health changes more enthusiastically, and had greater expectations of the possible results. It also indicated that using a variety of methods would be most effective, and that women wanted more options available to assist them in making changes.

At that time, I joined the Association of Humanistic Psychology (AHP), and attended my first National Conference. Many ideas, theories and questions that I had wondered about for years were awakened within me as I attended the panel discussions, workshops, and listened to the keynote speakers. I realized where the opportunities were for further research, and that it was imperative that I pursue them. I attended the AHP and National Institute for the Clinical Application of Behavioral Medicine (NICABM) conferences for many years. I have had the opportunity to take some interesting and informative workshops and to meet presenters who are researching and compiling the most recent research and the latest knowledge on the body/mind connections.

For the past 17 years, I have been in practice with two different Chiropractic offices working as a Neuromuscular Therapist, and I have private clients as well. I have a Masters in Communications and a Liberal Arts Bachelor Degree with minors in psychology, music and communications. While teaching as a university professor in communications, both interpersonal (public speaking) and intrapersonal (holistic courses) and working as a certified Neuromuscular Therapist, I decided to pursue a PhD. I wanted to do research in intrapersonal health communication.

For several years, I also voluntarily taught an Individual Development Course in the form of an 8-week Public Speaking class each fall for the Business and Professional Woman's Association (BPW) that is open to all women in the community for a nominal fee. It is designed to help develop public speaking skills, confidence and self-esteem for working women. I wrote a self-help manual on Impromptu Speaking, entitled "If I May Say" (Sprissler, 1998), as part of a Human Performance and Training class project. Although my training and studies were primarily in Interpersonal Communication, I became fascinated with Intrapersonal Communication (self-talk) and was starting to do some research in that area.

I attended and became certified in Dr. Bernie Siegel's Exceptional Cancer Treatment Program (ECaP). This is an interactive three-part training program for the development of a comprehensive framework for inspiring and motivating individuals to take an active and meaningful role in their healthcare.

I trained as an Arthritis Coping and Education (ACE) Group Leader, and became a member of the Arthritis Foundation's Speakers Bureau. I have facilitated both arthritis and fibromyalgia support groups. I have represented the arthritis foundation at many health fairs. I also conducted several workshops and seminars on holistic health issues and methodologies. All of my training and professional experiences, along with the doctorate research finally merged together. I therefore am sharing this with you in the hopes that as a practitioner, caregiver or patient you will gain insight into what conditions set us up for disease and chronic conditions. As well as analyzation and consideration of the paths to healthier living.

"Do not ask how, do not ask why, do not ponder the possibilities, or the nots. Just imagine, affirm, and plan. Dream and wish and say: Thank you. And it will be, and so it is."   *- Anon*

Prologue

Welcome to this book. I hope you will jump around, find information you need now, look up other things later when you're ready for them. It's about life – mine and yours. How to process what has happened so far. How to make plans and design your future health.

How's your life going? Mine is great. I've had lots of experiences. It's really quite exciting. I have known wonderful unexpected surprises, and some awful shocks. I have known deep love, happiness and some wealth. Also, hurt, loss and bereavement. Strangers who have opened their hearts and homes to me, and friends who have forsaken me.

Sound something like your life? I'll bet we share a lot of the same experiences. And that you have a lot others that are different from me. Isn't this interesting? Like a movie that the plot keeps getting deeper so that by now you can't count on it turning out any particular way. Especially when you plan on things going a certain way.

You can manage some of it, you know. Intention and positiveness brings it to you. Let go of all that is not serving you and try to stay in balance. If you have it, cherish it, use it, and share it. If you don't have it, develop all that you do have. It's more than enough to get you through.

The winner at life is the person who is the most satisfied, who has made the most personal growth. Who stepped out of the mould, made their own path, went the extra distance, gave up comfort and laziness to help another, knew how to cherish themselves, and gave what and when they could, and protected themselves when they had to. There are a gazillion books out there, which can be of enormous help to you. Please, go get a couple. Pick out the ones you're most likely to read and/or apply.

Here are some of the thoughts and questions that led to the development of this book:

An individual is living with the experience of a chronic painful condition, and despairs of feeling better and having a healthier lifestyle. While not immediately life threatening, the diagnosis carries the weight of major lifestyle changes with the possibility of curtailing of some activities. Often the individual has a "defeatist" attitude, and the mindset of succumbing to life as a semi-invalid. There are feelings of helplessness or depression, and an acceptance of the prognosis. Usually there is a lack of desire to seek out other opinions, or alternative health care options.

Yet many individuals do start to think about trying something to improve their situation. What intrapersonal communication (self-talk) took place to make this change in their thinking? I conducted a research study to examine what the change in that communication was, and how that change came to take place. I am continually learning about the physical and mental aspects of the body and the ways that they are truly integrated. I have studied the triggering agents and lifestyle choices for becoming ill, and the ability within each person to heal, even the most debilitating disease. I consider myself as a "holistic health coach" helping people through the healing journey.

Although the research study contained in this book focused on women suffering with fibromyalgia, the book is about anybody living with a painful or chronic condition. There are several methods and practices researched and presented in depth, but there are also many more available.

Over the years, I have listened as female clients, who are dealing with chronic conditions, especially fibromyalgia, tell me a similar story. They feel alone and misunderstood. They are fighting a battle every day to deal with pain, and yet try to appear somewhat normal to those around them. They complain that most of their family and friends think they are dramatizing their condition, or even neglecting themselves or responsibilities, because they do not understand the intensity of the client's afflictions.

These women also fall into similar life experiences. The largest group have husbands who are workaholics or travel a lot for work. Often, their symptoms improve to some degree when the husband is home for a few days, and deteriorate when he goes back on his regular schedule. Others have recently experienced an exhausting and terrible divorce, or have had a traumatic experience sometime in their life. Both groups feel lonely and abandoned. They believe they have no support system. They feel that their families both immediate and extended, feel sympathy for them but don't really understand. Those with children feel waves of emotional despair, as it is too painful to lift or hug their children. The children especially feel estranged, and do not realize how sensitive mother's skin is to any pressure at all.

And some days the women just don't care, and don't feel like trying to do anything. Yet, the more they lay there and center on their symptoms the worse they feel, and the more despair they realize. Several of the women have been told by their doctors and physical therapists that they have very limited wellness possibilities. That they should give up and accept, learn to live with, and adapt to your body as it is now. Coupled with a lot of day-to-day pain, and any "baggage" that they are carrying around, they became resigned. They now have the attitude and belief system that "this is as good as it gets". Often they almost "brag" about their degree of pain, and their pain threshold, seemingly proving how their physical problems are so much worse than other peoples.

Many researchers have explored fibromyalgia causes and medical, nutritional and complementary medicine approaches to alleviate symptoms, but little has been explored regarding the self-talk communication used to improve the condition. Nor, on the effectiveness of this information being used with fibromyalgia patients with severe symptoms, especially if they are also in a state of despair or depression.

As a holistic health professor and as a neuromuscular therapist, I work with a lot of clients with chronic conditions. Many questions regarding the progress of some of them were factored into the design of this book. I have found that frequently they get overwhelmed, depressed, are in too much pain, and/or are too weak to take the necessary steps to formulate a wellness program for themselves.

Possibilities are available for everyone who has a chronic disease or condition. The individual quality of life can be greatly improved, when the aches, pains and difficulties of the condition are alleviated, or in some cases, eliminated. There are many ways that an individual can use to begin travelling the path to self-healing. But what does the individual say to him/herself to get motivated to try one of them? What is needed to get up out of bed when he/she is so tired, and in pain, and depressed? What does he/she have to say to get dressed and not skip a chiropractic, massage therapy, or physical therapy session because he/she is overwhelmed by the effort of getting bathed, dressed and clothed? Or to begin a nutritional program, or do some mild exercising?

What does he/she have to say to him/herself in order to overcome the emotional baggage that Dr. Bernie Siegel and others say we carry around? The guilt, shame and blame and other damaging effects of the messages received so far in life? The baggage that allows her to become a welcome host for disease and chronic conditions. What gives her the inspiration to try Rubin Battino's or Bellaruth Naparstack's guided imagery, or biofeedback, or any of the many other effective therapies available? What does he/she have to say to start believing in the possibility of having a fulfilling and healthy life full of joy, for him/herself?

This book explores the diverse range of intrapersonal issues and processes, and also the importance of the type and degree of self-talk, self-scripting, self-monitoring and self-assessing. If we can learn to maintain positiveness in our lives, we allow ourselves to be open to growth possibilities and improving our physical and psychological well-being.

The study included herein addresses the ways to get through life by developing a balance of all of the aspects of total wellness, no matter what stage you may be at in the present. It presents the idea of being open to the possibility for creating ideal health through changes in thoughts, interpretations and choices. It shows that health is an optimal integration of our conscious mind, our body and the environment. Every experience we have is metabolized in the molecules which comprise our body. Thus, we are the way we perceive the world, which is the result of all past experiences. We change the quality of our body by changing the quality of our experience. Experience is the result of our perception, thus change perception, change experience, and we change our bodies. We change our perception by expansion of our consciousness. And thus, we come back to the importance of self-talk and the fact that everything within ourselves must be in balance for optimal total wellness.

This book is intended to bridge the gap between the many publications on possibilities and potentials of the self and the important information on the theories available today. The knowledge brought about from this study can help people to go inside themselves and find their inner resources to restore themselves where the mind is at peace with the healing processes that are taking place. The individual could then begin to formulate ideas and set goals for lifestyle changes to progress to a different physical state. Hopefully, it will help individuals to discard ideas of limitations and realize the unbound nature of self, to continue to practice actual physical evidence of these possibilities and then continue on their own path of continuous discovery. The last step is to support the process of reestablishing a healing balance that may be catalytic to an individual's innate healing faculties.

Alternative systems of medicine stress the interconnectedness of all things; and consciousness is seen as playing an integral role in the physical universe. There is no single cause for disease. Health and disease lie along a continuum and represent the degree of harmony with the universe. Integrative systems are essentially preventive, to help the individual preserve balance. They also offer the opportunity for self-responsibility; thus the individual can maintain a sense of power, of self-control and self-determination.

From the information gathered, could some techniques be developed from the commonality of all of the participants in this study that would benefit many? In my conversations with several medical doctors and practitioners, the same thread of concern arises. Many professionals are now convinced that integrative therapies work and that body/mind connectiveness is the basis for many healing techniques. Often, they are able to convince their patients. However, the hardest and sometimes impossible task is to get the patient to start. Could the results of this study then be used as a tool for those practitioners?

Integrative Medicine is becoming a widely accepted option for thousands of people. Many therapies are beginning to be recognized within mainstream medicine. Integrative/ Complementary health sessions are being prescribed by an increasing number of doctors, and several insurance companies are including coverage within their policies. Medicare has recently extended coverage for limited preventative treatments.

The discoveries within this book have social meaning and implications for women who are diagnosed with fibromyalgia and others living with chronic painful conditions. On a personal level, there is important information for the individual patient's family and friends. For the community as a whole, this information will benefit other women with the same diagnosis. This also extends to those in the medical communities who care for them. Although in order to conduct focused research, the study was conducted on women with fibromyalgia as one of the many chronic painful conditions patients are living with.

Fibromyalgia is a form of arthritis, however it attacks the soft tissue, rather than the bones or joints, and although it primarily affects the myofascia and muscles, there is a vast range of symptoms and areas of the body that can be affected. It is a syndrome that combines pain, fatigue, anxiety and depression. Because my experience with individuals living with a chronic condition and despairing of the ability of a healthier change has been 90% women, I decided to focus on women. I chose the minimum age of 35 and the maximum age of 65 as the ages when most women are diagnosed, have had enough experience to have lived with debilitating symptoms for some time, a lessor degree of aging complications, and have had at least a year of some improvement. To protect anonymity, I have given each of the women the name of a flower. After all, they have opened themselves up to a new way of living and coping and are growing more each day.

*"Knowing is not enough; we must apply.
Willing is not enough; we must do."*
- Johann Wolfgang von Goethe

Introduction: The Causes and Cures for Chronic Painful Conditions

Over our lifetime many ailments are the body's attempts to process intellectual and emotional energy. Grief in the lungs, anger in the liver, worry in the stomach and fright held in the kidneys are some of the ways the body attempts to clear emotional energy. When you are ill or imbalanced, treating your whole self rather than the physical self alone can enable you to determine the source of your sickness. Understanding that your physical symptoms may be an expression of emotional discomfort can help you form a balanced treatment regimen to ensure that you quickly recover whole health again.

Many of the ailments we experience over the course of our lives are the body's attempts to process intellectual and emotional energy. When you feel ill or imbalanced, treating your whole self rather than treating the physical self alone can empower you to determine the root cause of sickness. Since you understand that your physical symptoms may be an expression of emotional discomfort, you can establish a balanced treatment regimen to ensure that you quickly recover your good health.

Talbot (2007) points out that medical researchers have known for more than sixty years that chronic or repeated bouts of stress will lead to a shrinking of the thymus gland (one of the key immune tissues in the body) and to a general suppression of immune-system strength. We know that cortisol has a direct effect on shrinking the thymus and inhibiting white blood cell production and activity. Cortisol suppresses the ability of white blood cells to secrete chemical messengers (interleukins and interferons), so the different varieties of immune-system cells become unable to communicate with each other in a way that would allow them to more effectively fight off infections.

Cortisol can actually act as a signal to many immune-system cells to simply shut off and stop working (that is, the cells die). During periods of chronic stress, cortisol levels remain elevated and immune-system integrity begins to suffer. The chronically stimulated immune-system cells start to break down, losing their ability to fight off invading pathogens. In some cases they can start to unleash their destructive properties on the body's own tissues, resulting in a variety of allergies, as well as in autoimmune diseases such as multiple sclerosis, lupus, fibromyalgia, and rheumatoid arthritis. And, obesity, heart disease, diabetes, depression/anxiety, Alzheimer's disease, osteoporosis, suppressed libido, frequent colds/flu/infection, and memory/concentration problems are all linked to stress.

But what is stress? Can you see it or touch it? We hear so much about stress and stressors, especially how it affects us. But what does that really mean? Stress is a response to any threat or perception of threat that promotes the idea that something necessary for well-being is going to be taken away. Each stress event is experienced in the present, but has its resonance from the past. The psyche is the brain center that perceives, interprets emotional stimuli and processes emotional responses, which affect the nervous system, the endocrine glands and the immune system. It is necessary to be aware when we are experiencing stress and to express our emotions effectively to assert our needs and to maintain the integrity of our emotional boundaries. These should conform to our present needs and not to unconscious, unsatisfied needs from the past. And to provide for those needs rather than repressing them. Awareness also means learning what the signs of stress are in our bodies and how our bodies let us know when our minds have missed the signs.

At first glance, many of us might view the close relationship between stress, cortisol, and the long list of chronic diseases as a hopeless disaster just waiting to happen—and for a great many people, it is. However, armed with the right information and the proper motivation, we can do a great deal to counteract these potential problems. The general idea is to manage the stress response in such a way that cortisol levels are maintained within their optimal range - not too high and not too low - with long-term health and wellness as the outcome.

Another reason is that autoimmune disorders can be a viral or bacterial infection, although a faulty gene may also be present. Viruses and bacteria can devise ways of hiding deep within the immune system. Often the result of antibiotics which were either not strong enough or not completing a course of therapy. Bacteria mutates and becomes resistant to future treatment. Extreme or unrelenting stress increases secretions and activates B-cells to produce antibodies. Many people will claim that their disease began after the death of a loved one or a seriously stressful event. We are also exposed the antibiotics that are fed to beef, poultry and farm-grown fish which we then ingest.

This book is about the effects of attitude and illness, and the use of various methods to aid in healing. The focus is on living with and easing chronic conditions, although the applications and explanations are beneficial to anyone dealing with pain.

A research study was conducted on 14 women with fibromyalgia, and the results showed the impact of positive and negative self-talk and the explanation of how each impact the body at a bio-cellular level. It explains how using the right tools to create a positive emotion can release beneficial chemicals to help heal at a cellular level.

Why do some people get sick or develop chronic conditions? Why do some people choose to try to get better? Why do people get better in spite of the seriousness of their condition, or a negative prognosis? This book endeavors to answer these questions and to look at the experience of women living with a chronic painful condition who have been improving their health. What in their experiences and mindsets led to their improved conditions? Although there is no known cause or cure for fibromyalgia there are theories regarding what may lead up to it, and methods or options patients can use to improve their condition. But looking at a comparable concept, what may be the causes and the cures for fibromyalgia and other chronic conditions?

Perhaps the following examples will help us to understand the limited lifestyle of those living with chronic conditions and/or chronic pain:

Deborah arises in the morning, visits the bathroom, and lies down again to rest. She then struggles to take a shower, and then has to rest. Later she gets dressed, and after resting again, attempts to make an easy breakfast for herself. After putting away the food, and leaving the dishes in the sink she lies down to take a nap. She is exhausted. Several hours later she will arise again and try to get on with her day.

Helen tries to help her husband and children off to work and school, meanwhile within she is screaming in pain. Her pain level throughout the day goes up and down, often crippling her. She cannot tolerate her children giving her a hug, or consoling them in her arms when they hurt themselves. The pain level is too strong.

These are examples of the millions of people dealing every day with a painful state of health. This book is about patients dealing with a chronic state of health, and in particular, those living with painful conditions. It is based on a research study I conducted with women who are living with fibromyalgia. Although the women mentioned above are severe cases, almost all fibromyalgia patients have to alter their lifestyle somewhat to manage their health. This is true for most people living with a chronic health problem.

This book is based on a narrative based phenomenological and qualitative study and includes analysis of the commonalties of themes of in-depth interviews with women who have been diagnosed with fibromyalgia, and have realized an improved state in their condition for at least a year. It explores the approach participants used to realize this state and the self-communication with themselves that led to that positive change.

Based on these interviews the following themes and sub-themes emerged:

- Comorbid conditions
- Lack of trust
- Self-care
- Inner strength
- Alternative therapies
- Perseverance

The women were asked open-ended questions and allowed to speak freely regarding their experience of living with fibromyalgia. Treatments and remedies were varied, as they each realized they would have to find their own pain relief and change their attitude about the disease. They were all persistent and creative. Most of them adopted one or more of the methodologies covered herein without realizing it. The study also explored how attitude and belief system changes can modify health at the bio-cellular level. The research study can be used as a basis for further narrative research. It is of interest to women suffering with fibromyalgia, and the medical practitioners and therapists who care for them.

This book shows how people get sick. How negative emotions release negative chemicals which affect us at a cellular level. It also reveals how people can heal. People get sick because negative emotions such as fear, anger, anxiety, and negative stressors, cause glands such as the pituitary, endocrine and adrenal glands to produce harmful chemicals such as dopamine, adrenaline, and cortisol that enter and weaken the cells.

Health improves because positive emotions and exercises, such as prayer, laughter and meditation, result in the production of calming and healing chemicals such as melatonin and seratonin, to name a few. There is also a necessity to manage stress, create an emotional balance and set a goal, to be detailed, realistic, and to set criteria for success. The interrelationship between our experiences, feelings, and body chemistry are intricate. Specific mental states effect specific glandular secretions, circulatory patterns, and organ functions. Therefore, there is probably no limit to the influencing of function and behavior by feelings and attitudes.

This book will present selected mind/body practices such as Neurolinguistic Programming (NLP), Psychoneuroimmunology (PNI), Focusing, Intrapersonal Communication, the significance of placebos and examine fibromyalgia as one of the chronic painful conditions that many patients are living with day to day.

Accountability, self-efficacy, changing attitudes and belief systems all play a part in turning around chronic conditions and illness. Often, one must fool their mind in order to enlist their own powers of self-healing.

Using placebos, hypnosis, autosuggestion, faith healing, visualization, and/or positive thinking, one can begin to control their health. Along with being creative in putting forth the effort and seeking various treatment methods and lifestyle changes. If one agrees to make choices that equate with joy, satisfaction, and trust, then a positive physiological response occurs throughout the body, particularly in the immune system.

Why do people get sick? Why do people get better? It is necessary to formulate an individual and diverse treatment plan.

The study explored the fibromyalgia experience through interviews with women who have an improved health and quality of life. It was conducted through audio taped personal interviews with the participants narrating their experiences. The descriptive data were analyzed using a grounded theory technique. The effects of the individual's type of self-talk and the results of that self-talk on the overall on-going, improved condition of the individual was investigated to demonstrate that the mind is part of the healing process. This study looks at the intra-personal communication (self-talk) aspect of treating chronic conditions or diseases, in this case, fibromyalgia.

The study was conducted to obtain a detailed picture of the way in which a number of people, who are living with a chronic physical condition and have improved their health to some degree, interpret their experience. It is an attempt to get the "lived" experience through involved and well-documented methods and practices, beginning with extensive open-ended, unstructured interviews.

What self-messages enable one person to search for solutions to improve their medical condition, and another person to identify with their illness and give up? What intrapersonal communication will change the belief that their health and lifestyle is not going to change? What types of intrapersonal communication took place among those fibromyalgia patients who have improved?

Deep intrapersonal communication to promote healing is more than affirmations. What types of processes are used to help the individual learn to maintain positiveness in their life, and to allow him/herself to be open to growth possibilities, and improving his/her physical and psychological well-being? Would knowledge of the processes followed by those who have improved their health help others who are "stuck" in a despairing state of ill-health?

These questions are answered in the following chapters.

"The only way of finding the limits of the possible is by going beyond them into the impossible."
-Arthur C. Clarke

Chapter 1. Chronic Conditions and Quality of life

How does disease start? According to Jones (2010) we put poisons in our bodies to get rid of cancer. We take medications that interrupt our body's natural chemistry. We cut out organs from our bodies, causing other organs to work harder. We don't have cures, just possible maintenance for many chronic conditions. Each disease begins with a soul discovery. The way you operate in life marked by your feelings, attitudes and beliefs, combined with the lessons your soul came to earth to learn, determine your risk for contracting a disease.

The onset of disease is made up of four emotional sufferings:
- *Lack of self-love* – emotional eruptions can especially undermine health if absent. Love is the universal energy that sustains life. Self-love is the energy that sustains the body.
- *Powerlessness* – when you feel like a victim your energy gets zapped and you're at risk of your immune system collapsing and waiting for a serious trigger event, giving you no chance to escape serious consequences.

- *Resentment* – pent up from negative experiences builds pressure in our bodies, which can turn to anger or rage under the surface.
- *Anger* - which can turn to rage when suppressed, can erupt the triggers for the growth of cancer cells or other symptoms.

A healthy body, with self-love as its foundation, releases anger and resentment every time they come up so they don't build up pressure and spark symptoms, conditions, or disease. Pressures from these emotional sufferings build pressure in our bodies. If not released or resolved, every time they come up, over time they can develop into anger or rage under the surface. The feeling of powerlessness can suppress or even collapse one's immune system, contributing to the development of disease. Immense power is yours when you take full responsibility for yourself and reclaim it. A healthy body always keeps its personal power, never sinking into victim mode. It knows there's a solution to every problem, perhaps even with professional help to find it.

Possibilities are available for everyone who has a chronic disease or condition. The individual's quality of life can be greatly improved when the aches, pains, and difficulties of the condition are alleviated, or in some cases, eliminated. There are many pathways that an individual can use to begin travelling the path to self-healing. But what does the individual say to herself to get motivated to try one of them? What is needed to get up out of bed when a woman is so tired, and in pain, and depressed? What does she have to say to get dressed and not skip a chiropractic, massage therapy, or physical therapy session because she is overwhelmed by the effort of getting bathed, dressed and clothed? Or to begin a nutritional program, or do some mild exercising?

Elevated symptoms of depression are quite common in people with chronic pain and serve to exacerbate the aversive aspects of pain, according to a study conducted by Vowles, MacLaren and Gross (2006). Recent analyses have suggested that some portion of treatment completers do not show a significant reduction in symptoms of depression following treatment and, therefore, continue to experience strong levels of distress and disability. Results showed that individuals with consistently high symptoms were more distressed and disabled before and after psychosocial and cognitive treatment compared with their counterparts.

Given that individuals with consistent symptoms of depression appear to improve to a lesser degree over the course of treatment, accurate identification and the provision of appropriate treatment will be important areas for future work. Such an approach will likely require the field in general to move away from focusing merely on the form of intensity of symptoms, to the function that they serve or impact that they have on patient behavior.

Zautra, et al. (2007) conducted a study examining the role of past episodes of depression on pain reports for patients with rheumatoid arthritis. Patients were evaluated by a rheumatologist and then asked to report joint and bodily pain throughout the study. Patients with a history of two or more episodes of major depression had more pain as baseline, and exhibited higher pain in response to the stress induction than did patients with either only one episode or no history of depression. Such findings provide a new insight in the dynamic relationships between depression, stress, and pain.

What does a woman with fibromyalgia have to say to herself in order to overcome the emotional baggage that Dr. Bernie Siegel (2002) and others say one carries around? Such as the guilt, shame, blame, and other damaging effects of the messages received so far in life? Or to overcome the negative baggage that allows her to become a welcome host for disease and chronic conditions? What gives her the inspiration to try guided imagery, or biofeedback, or any of the many other effective therapies available? What does she have to say to herself to start believing in the possibility of having a fulfilling and healthy life full of joy for herself? Siegel (2003) also states that healing one's life is a gift that everyone can appreciate, and a cure may be the result, even if it is not the primary goal. "I try to get people to reclaim their lives, to live, rather than trying to avoid dying. …We also have to remember that we have our intellect and our intuition, or unconscious, at work. We need to know how they both react to our disease and therapeutic choices" (pp. 13-14).

    This research was conducted because of the belief in the importance of individual intrapersonal communication. I am interested in the diverse range of intrapersonal issues and processes, and also the importance of the type and degree of self-talk, self-scripting, self-monitoring, and self-assessing. I know that if one can learn to maintain positiveness in their lives that they allow themselves to be open to growth possibilities and improving their physical and psychological well-being.

    This study addresses the ways to get through life by developing a balance of all of the aspects of total wellness, no matter what stage one may be at in the present. It presents the idea of being open to the possibility for creating ideal health through changes in thoughts, interpretations, and choices. It shows that health is an optimal integration of the conscious mind, the body, and the environment.

    Complementary and Alternative Medicine (CAM) has received increased attention in mainstream medicine since 1993, according to Chan (2008). It has become clear the users of CAM are not primarily dissatisfied with conventional care, but have a more holistic approach to health or simply appreciate multiple treatment options. "What was once identified as 'alternative medicine' has become 'complementary', 'holistic', and 'integrative'. The demarcation between CAM and mainstream medicine continues to shift" (pp. 2685-2686).

Although the definition of integrative, complementary, and alternative medicine remains under discussion, according to Salkeld (2008), the medical literature contains few reports on the process of integration of CAM methods into clinical practice. The introduction of CAM modalities into practice allows physicians to address body, mind, emotional, and spiritual causes of disease. Incorporation of CAM modalities into clinical practice by biomedically trained physicians with additional CAM experience gave them flexibility to offer patients different treatment options and alleviated the need to reconcile conflicting theories of disease etiology.

The following chapters present the historical progression of theories and practices in mind/body medicine and methods for self-healing. It depicts the progression of physical disorders and expounds upon the theories of 1) how people get sick, 2) acknowledge their illness, and 3) endeavor to improve their physiology. The research shows the ways people can heal, and provides an understanding how lifestyle affects human physiology and the options open to make changes to effect healing.

These sections build on previous research and studies over the years, and show how medical science has progressed, and the outlook for further research in these areas. The theories and techniques of intrapersonal communication, focusing, placebo response, and psychoneuroimmunology are reviewed. The condition of fibromyalgia is also reviewed in depth.

"The greatest revolution of our generation is the discovery that human beings, by changing the inner attitudes of their minds, can change the outer aspects of their lives."
    -William James, psychologist, philosopher

Chapter 2. Intra-Personal Communication: Self-talk for Self-health

To understand intrapersonal communication or self-talk, one must first understand the role of the brain in conceptualizing and understanding intrapersonal communication. As will be explained, several disciplines interplay to realize a communication perspective on intrapersonal communication and on the specific interhemispheric and intermodular processes inherent in intrapersonal communication. Stacks and Andersen (1989) stated that for more than 100 years, studies focused on the "dominant" left hemisphere of the brain, but in the late 1960s and through the 1970s the right hemisphere's role was explored. They showed the right hemisphere's role as being *dominant* for many nonverbal functions. The left hemisphere was viewed as *dominant* for many verbal functions. Motor functioning of the right side of the body is controlled by the left hemisphere, and left-side functioning is controlled by the right hemisphere. The brain is now hypothesized to work as an organized whole, and the idea of a *holistic* brain has evolved. This brain requires input from both hemispheres to *process* and ultimately *interpret* the world surrounding its owner.

They also explain that about the same time, communication researchers began to express an interest in the processing abilities of the brain. The intent was to understand how and why the human being communicated, and the nature of the message system underlying communication. The brain was considered to have different modules or centers, each interdependent upon the other for processing. Research pointed to the importance of understanding how the brain communicated with itself as the beginning point of communication or as *neurocommunication.* Interaction among brain modules may be a true form of intrapersonal communication.

Another term is interhemispheric communication, which is the transmission of messages between hemispheres or modules, that is, a distinct intrapersonal communication process. Thus, intrapersonal communication covers many disciplines, including, but not limited to: psychology and its many branches, neurophysiology, sociology, and the various kinds of communication. Studies in communications show that intrapersonal communication includes emotional reasoning, "should" statements, personalization or self-blame, and labeling. This is done through internal dialogue, visualization, beliefs, and assumptions.

When one controls these factors, one can carry out a variety of tasks and activities, both physical and mental, more successfully. As an example, self-talk training improves one's performance. Mental imaging improves decision making, strategy formulation, and other complex skills. Managing one's beliefs and assumptions helps one deal with destructive habits, phobias, depression, and other dysfunctions. It is important that an individual engage in an ever-constant dialogue with him/herself in order to influence his/her behavior, feelings, self-esteem and stress level. The structure of the unconscious processing with the addition of significant information into the intrapersonal communication system brings self-talk to a level of awareness.

Rethinking and reverbalizing these inner dialogues allows one a better chance to improve these factors. For instance, consider the relationship between self-talk and emotional issues. Treadwell and Kendall (1996) conducted a study among therapists regarding "the use of self-talk as a gauge for recognizing their own and their client's cognitive distortions and ability to manage anxiety, and the relationship between self-talk and therapy process variables" (pp. 941-949). The study showed that negative self-statements related to childhood anxiety disorders and their treatment and their improvement. As anxious distress is reduced, the accompanying negative self-talk becomes less frequent.

Self-talk, both positive and negative, plays an equal role in the emotion of anger (Newman & Peterson, 1996). In their study adult women survivors of incest were compared to other women with respect to questionnaire measures of manifest anger. The use of self-talk was measured, both positive and negative, in regard to this anger. The results showed that incest survivors were angrier than other women were, both in general and with their parents. Anger toward mother and anger toward father were comparable.

Next, is the relationship between stress and self-talk. According to Epstein, Seymour and Katz (1992) stress, whether externally or internally produced, is associated with emotional symptoms. "Coping abilities via intrapersonal communication determine positive or negative emotions. Daily stressors consist largely of self-produced stressors. Total stress was significantly associated with a wide range of symptom variables, but most strongly associated with emotional symptoms." (pp. 813-825) The importance of the awareness of, and the management of self-talk in relation to individual perception of the self has been studied (Bunce, Scott, Larsen & Peterson, 1995). Traumatized college students reported more trait anxiety and lower self-esteem than did nontraumatized students. They scored higher on neuroticism, were more introverted, and were less emotionally stable than nontraumatized participants studied.

Gesell (2007) describes self-talk as the "ongoing dialogue people have with themselves that determines their behavior. Self-talk reflects and creates individual's emotional states so when the self-talk is negative individuals become more stressed, less confident, and more concerned with other people's opinions. In addition, people tend to believe their self-talk is real and objective, and are not always aware that it comes from a feeling or belief that they have" (pp. 20-21). Another way to look at self-talk is as the expression of what people believe is true about a situation. There are many forms of negative self-talk including awfulizing, catastrophizing, overgeneralizing, polarized thinking, and shoulding (Gesell, 2007).

Benson and Proctor (2003) say that is it necessary to sever your consciousness completely from negative "mental tape recordings." This change of inner direction will automatically turn on an inner switch, which will enable you to generate regular breakouts and peak experiences that can transform your entire life. Although this basic trigger mechanism may appear simple, the process is actually rooted in complex biochemical interaction that occur throughout the brain and elsewhere in the body.

These studies document both the opportunities and the difficulties involved in analyzing intrapersonal communication. They highlight many of the concepts and questions that arise, and present a variety of topics, disciplines, and arguments. They reflect the complexities and confusion of where intrapersonal communication fits, and the difficulty of approaching it from only a communication standpoint. What is needed is some theory or research result that specifies how intrapersonal communication affects different individuals in different situations using a diversified, interdisciplinary approach.

While some of these questions are answered in the literature, additional views would add to the diversity of the knowledge. Also, new information may augment previous findings in the light of the changing communications environment, thus further demonstrating the importance of self-talk and self-healing and the importance of psychoneuroimmunology. Some of the findings reported here have substantiated these connections.

Three areas maximize the activity of the naturally occurring self-healing capability according to Jahnke (1999). The first is the choice of attitudes and mental influences. When one chooses to think, believe, and act from a position of power, refusing to be a victim of circumstances, the healer within is automatically strengthened. The second area of choice is lifestyle. From moment to moment, one elects whether to enhance or sabotage the healer within through their behaviors and personal choices. The third area of choice is personal self-care, the practice of self-healing and health enhancement methods. The interaction of these three choice areas has become the foundation of health care and healing deep into the 21st century.

The research results of Pert (1997) have provided evidence of the biochemical basis for awareness and consciousness. Perception and awareness can change physiology and neurology and create an entirely new body. This transformation takes place over a network linking all of the systems and organs, engaging all of the molecules of emotion, as the means of communication. These molecules of emotion run every system in the body, and this communication system is in effect a demonstration of the body-mind's intelligence. This is an intelligence that is wise enough to seek wellness, and one that can potentially keep us healthy and disease free without the modern high-tech medical interventions one now relies on. Intrapersonal communication is a determinant factor of effectiveness of mental and emotional states on the immune system.

Psychoneuroimmunology is one of the most important disciplines in studying the interaction of mind and body. Sivik (2000) explains that interaction between the factors involved in the preservation of life is always involved in the development of all kinds of diseases. A balanced interaction between the different memory and communication systems of the human organism is necessary for the preservation of health, and disturbances in these communication systems underlie the developments of disease.

In order for the human organism to be prepared for and able to adequately adapt to change, it must be able to preserve stability in spite of demands and strain. This allostatic state can only be achieved if the communication between the different behavioral and emotional systems is unimpeded and adequate. It is essential that the different fields of psychosomatic medicine are not divided by their different subdisciplines and variety of focus, but rather it is crucial that they are bonded together into one strong multifaceted and comprehensive paradigm.

According to Roberts (2000) symptoms arise in the area of the body that is the weakest link in the person's mind-body system. Symptoms are stored physiological expressions of emotional and psychological areas of distress, related to the person's unique life narrative. Understanding where symptoms are stored, how the client experiences them, and the meaning the symptoms have to the client, helps our understanding of incorporating mind-body approaches to best formulate interventions to help our clients heal.

This study will contribute to the scope of research in intrapersonal health communications using several methods. Presenting and understanding the role of intrapersonal communication in the healing process, conducting an intensive study of specific phenomena in relation to how they have been used by the participating individuals, and by the narration of their particular experiences.

"I believe we create every so-called illness in our body. The body, like everything else in life, is a mirror of our inner thoughts and beliefs. The body is always talking to us, if we will only take the time to listen. Every cell within your body responds to every single thought you think and every word you speak."
- Louise Hay

Chapter 3. Examining the Methods and Procedures

Focusing

Evans (2006) states that when the body is placed in an almost constant state of alert, the adrenal glands become tired eventually which leads to a depleted and panicky state, rather than stimulated and awake. Change happens when one feels more in one's body than one can cognitively understand. An exploration into the concept of focusing is important to the study of intrapersonal communication.

Listening and focusing are invaluable skills for self-communication and for reducing stress. They provide new opportunities for individuals to take better care of themselves (Klagsbrun, 2001). Gendlin (1999) theorized that when an individual goes past words and rational explanations he or she can attain new levels of awareness within the body. It is on this level that real change occurs.

Hendricks (2007) says that experiential psychotherapy originated in Gendlin's "Philosophy of the Implicit". Some of its main concepts are bodily felt sense, fresh emergence of words from the felt sense, and carrying forward the implicit with small steps of change. Successful clients pay attention to their experiences in a specific way. They pay attention to what is, at first, a vague yet persistent, bodily felt sense of some problem or situation. They often create a metaphor to describe it. "When they find words or an image that 'gets it exactly', there is a felt relief and sense of meaning and movement. Success correlated not with the content but with the manner in which the client discusses these contents" (p. 271).

The therapeutic relationship is described as a curative factor in its own right as well as being facilitative for other tasks according to Leijssen (2007). Experiential tasks that facilitate working on the intrapsychic, interpersonal, and existential domains are distinguished. Clearing space helps clients find a right distance for exploring their experience when they are too close or too distanced from their emotions. Interpersonal work takes the lead when maladaptive interactional patterns are hindering the relational life of the client. Metacommunicative feedback and interpersonal experiences in the therapeutic encounter act as an invitation to develop new ways of communicating. Existential processes are challenged when the client struggles with the givens of life. Finally, the "inner guide" found in accessing experiencing may involve an awareness of a transcendent dimension that leads one to spiritual growth.

The basis of Focusing is that the mind and body are intimately connected and that by listening to the body one comes to understand one's self (Hinterkopf). Cornell (1996) believes that focusing occurs exactly at the interface of body-mind and consists of specific steps. The body sense is vague at first but will open up into words or images and an individual will experience a "felt shift" in his or her body. The individual will learn to live in a deeper place than just thoughts or feelings. Then the theory is that the content looks different and new solutions arise.

Klagsbrun (2001) explains the importance of focusing and the need to use it by describing it as follows. The body knows the world in a way that is distinctly different and separate from the way we know the world in our minds. Focusing is a way of gaining access to the body's experience of meaning and the individual moves from a whole *felt sense* of an experience to achieve a bodily resolution of that issue. She also states that a person is familiar with a body feeling that is connected directly to something that has happened in one's life: butterflies in the stomach before a performance review, or a tense feeling in the throat when one needs to share difficult news. Focusing involves spending time with a bodily sensation that is not yet clear and cannot really be put into words but that one feels has a connection to some issue or event in their life. It involves becoming a friend to one's own inner experience.

Focusing can be the inner compass that helps people navigate through the territory of serious illness (Klagsbrun, 2001). She explains that it encourages people to connect with body, mind, and spirit. It helps them to perceive inner messages and meanings rather than taking cues from others. And to understand their own stories in a fresh way in order to change unhealthy behaviors and to integrate the illness experience in such a way that one's humanity as a patient is expanded (Klagsbrun, 2001).

Iberg (1991) further explains focusing as enabling people to communicate effectively with themselves, in order to gain a deeper and more meaningful understanding of what they are feeling in the moment. Originally developed as a tool for the psychology field, focusing is being incorporated in healthcare by nurses, physicians, physical therapists, massage therapists, acupuncturists, and administrators, as well as individuals living with illness.

Although it is often used as a tool by these professionals, focusing can be taught to anyone and can be used by individuals. Most people learn best in focusing partnerships (NICABM, 2001).

According to the research shown herein, I believe that there are meanings beyond awareness that lead to emotional disturbance, physical illness, and spiritual distress. Focusing is a gentle, body-centered process that is used to access inner meanings; thus potentially bringing clarity to one's life issues. Therefore, it can be an important intrapersonal communication tool for healing.

"I identified in a very deep way with the individuals I was writing about because the theme that runs through this story is of extraordinary physical hardship and the will to overcome it. The owner, the jockey and the horse were all dealing with afflictions and nobody would have ever predicted that they would win one race, much less the Triple Crown. That is the fundamental struggle of my life, trying to get over this extremely devastating physical condition. The only time that I wasn't thinking about dealing with my physical suffering was when I was working on this book.
  - Laura Hillenbrand, author of 'Seabiscuit'

Psychoneuroimmunology (PNI)

Psychoneuroimmunology is the study of the interaction between psychological processes and the nervous and immune systems of the human body. PNI takes an interdisciplinary approach, incorporating psychology, neuroscience, immunology, physiology, pharmacology, molecular biology, psychiatry, behavioral medicine, infectious diseases, endocrinology, and rheumatology.

The main interests of PNI are the interactions between the nervous and immune systems and the relationships between mental processes and health. PNI studies, among other things, the physiological functioning of the neuroimmune system in health and disease; disorders of the neuroimmune system (autoimmune diseases; hypersensitivities; immune deficiency); and the physical, chemical and physiological characteristics of the components of the neuroimmune system in vitro, in situ, and in vivo. Neuroscience and immunology developed independently for many years, as explained by Ziemssen and Kern (2007).

Psychoneuroimmunology is a relatively new field that investigates interactions between behavior and the immune system, mediated by the endocrine and nervous systems. PNI research has demonstrated the immune regulatory mechanisms are part of a complex network of adaptive responses. This new knowledge holds considerable promise for expanding our understanding of the mechanisms underlying health and illness, and the role emotions and stress play in this equation. Behavioral interventions that reduce anxiety or distress decrease the intensity or duration of neuroendocrine responses, thereby effecting a change in immune function that promotes wellness and recovery from disease.

Folk wisdom has long suggested that stressful events take a toll on health. (Glaser & Kiecolt-Glaser, 2005). PNI is now providing key mechanistic evidence about the ways in which stressors - and the negative emotions that they generate – can be translated into physiological changes. PNI researchers have used animal and human models to learn how the immune system communicates bidirectionally with the central nervous and endocrine systems and how these interactions impact on health (p. 243).

Tausk, Elenkov and Moynihan (2008) assert that PNI is an evolving area of science that will help us understand the relationship between the mind and the body. The past 30 years of research in the field have validated the close relationship between the central nervous system and the immune system, and that stress modifies the delicate balance between health and disease. Seeking alternative interventions can only enhance our ability to treat patients. (pp. 22-

31) Glaser and Kiecolt-Glaser (2005) explain how stress is assessed as the following: "When events or environmental demands exceed an individual's ability to cope, the ensuing psychological stress response typically includes negative thoughts and emotions" (p. 243). These might include the number and types of recent significant stressful life changes, or the frequency of not controlling important things in life.

The psychological and immunological responses of individuals who are experiencing a distress-generating event or a more chronic stressor are associated with immune alterations. Stressors that are perceived as unpredictable and/or uncontrollable might continue to be associated with increased levels of stress hormones, even after repeated exposures. The ability to unwind after stressful events – to return to one's neuroendocrine baseline in a relatively short time – is thought to influence the total burden that stressors place on an individual (Glaser & Kiecolt-Glaser, 2005).

The Jensen and Patterson (2007) review identified 13 published controlled articles that evaluated the efficacy of hypnosis for the treatment of chronic pain. The findings indicated that "hypnosis interventions consistently produced significant decreases in pain associated with a variety of chronic pain problems. Also hypnosis was generally found to be more effective than nonhypnotic interventions such as attention, physical therapy, and education. Most of the hypnosis interventions for chronic pain include instructions in self-hypnosis" (pp. 275-287).

Battino (2000) presents a review of the scientific evidence for the effectiveness of mind/body work; a stimulus in the present calls forth in all dimensions the experiences from your past, which were triggered by the stimulus. He states that recent studies show that new nerve cells can be formed in the adult human brain. Factors that enhance the growth of new nerve cells are an enriched environment by which the brain is challenged with new information, and novel experiences and puzzles to be solved, and by physical exercise. Research is continuing in this area for its potential for better treatments for neurological diseases, but this work also emphasizes the importance of mind/body/environment interactions. Research in PNI and related areas have provided the missing scientific foundation for mind/body healing. If miserable and stressful thoughts can harm the body, then relaxation and happy thoughts can both heal and cure the body.

Psychoneuroimmunology is a part of behavioral medicine that has undergone explosive growth in recent years. It is an interdisciplinary field concerned with the integration of behavioral and biomedical science knowledge and techniques relevant to health and disease and the application of this knowledge and these techniques to prevention, treatment, and rehabilitation.

Ader (1981) asks if grief, depression, or anxiety can alter the ability to resist infections, allergies, autoimmunities or even cancer. The endocrine glands can influence the development, maintenance, and functions of the lymphocytes, which are the cells that subserve the immunologic functions. The hormones of the adrenal glands could promote lysis (the destruction or breakdown of one cell or microorganism) by a specific agent. Stress could also cause lysis of lymphocytes and thymic involution and great changes in lymphoid tissues.

Physicians, scientists, and lay people have suspected for thousands of years that the "mind"/nervous system influences the "body's" condition of health and its response to disease. In the mid-1920s serious and consistent attempts were made in the laboratory to pin down this phenomenon, according to Metal'nikov (1934). He documented that immune responses are common to both invertebrates and vertebrates and more importantly, that several immune reactions could be induced, in the absence of antigens, by classical conditioning techniques. This was the first clear experimental evidence of neuroimmunomodulation, the influence of the central nervous system upon general immune responses.

Ader (1981) explains that immunomodulation (NIM) and neuroimmunogenesis (NIG) can be divided roughly into three categories: psychic, neurophysiologic, and cellular-molecular. The psychic evidence for NIM had accumulated from experiments in stress conditioning, hypnosis, biological psychiatry, psychosomatic medicine, biofeedback and clinical observations of changes in immune responses associated with various affective disorders. Neurophysiologic regards the thinking that the immune system and the nervous system control each other.

Ader further explains that the best way to understand the way the brain can influence immune function involves hormones that are under control of the hypothalamic-pituitary axis. This directly controls the secretion of all known pituitary tropic hormones including those that act indirectly through the target glands: adrenal, thyroid, and gonads; or on target tissues: growth hormone and prolactin. He explains that brain modulation of the immune response possibly is mediated by direct secretion of brain peptides into the general circulation.

In addition to neuropeptides, several other biologic activities occur. These include endothelial (lining of the cell body) growth factor and brain growth factor. Another neurosecretion is melatonin, which is released into the blood. A fourth potential mechanism of neuroendrocrine modulation of the immune response is by way of the peripheral nervous system. It can secrete a variety of neuroregulatory peptides including somatostatin and vasoactive intestinal peptide. And a fifth way the brain could modulate the immune response is through behavior and autonomic regulation that are closely linked to neuroendrocrine mechanisms. These include changes in nutrition, altered circadian (sleep) rhythms (24 hour cycle of repetition such as sleeping and eating), vascular problems, elevated or depressed body temperature, and abnormal sleep/wake cycles.

Ader further states that the possible sites of action of any or all of the above mechanisms are potentially as complex as the immune system itself. Thus, the basic mechanisms by which the brain communicates biochemically or hormonally with the non-neuronal components are complex.

Neuroendrocrine cells acting through the system modulate a vast array of peripheral metabolic and hormonal systems. Within the body are three subsystems all concerned with maintaining this equilibrium, and each highly complex in itself. These are the nervous, endocrine and immune systems. The interaction between these three is intrinsically fascinating and highly relevant to disease. PNI is based on the idea that one's state of mind (psyche) initiates activities through the nervous system that have an effect on the immune system.

The most transformative scientific finding that confirmed the presence of the healer within was when Pert and her team at the National Institutes for Health (NIH) found that the body produces its own pain medication internally (Pert, 1997). These chemicals, called neurotransmitters or "information substances," are literally the biochemistry of thought and feelings. This validated the ancient Chinese idea that one actually produces a healing elixir within.

But how do one's thoughts and emotions actually affect their health? How do the messages that one receives and the dialogues that one conducts with themselves translate into physical and psychological changes within? The research and discussion up to this point has been the acceptance that a placebo, whatever its shape and source can indeed effect changes within oneself.

The subsequent paragraphs are an encapsulated version of Pert's research on psychoneuroimmunology, which will help to explain how physiological changes take place and the influence of one's intrapersonal communications and placebos that stimulate them are connected.

Pert's research (2002) reveals the body's internal chemicals, the neuropeptides and their receptors, are the actual biological underpinnings of our awareness, manifesting themselves as one's emotions, beliefs, and expectations, and profoundly influencing how one responds to and experiences their world, and forming an information network within the body. This is key to understanding how mind and body are interconnected and how emotions can be manifested throughout the body.

Consciousness has come up in the context of studying pain and the role of opiate receptors and endorphins in modulating pain. ...The area called periaqueductal gray, located around the third ventricle of the brain, is filled with opiate receptors, making it a kind of control area for pain. This area is also loaded with receptors for virtually all the neuropeptides that have been studied.

There are some people who do not perceive pain, depending on how they structure their experience. These people are able to plug into their periaqueductal gray with their consciousness and set pain thresholds. The person has an experience that brings with it pain, but a part of the person consciously does something so that the pain is not felt. ...It is possible to conceive of mind and consciousness as an emanation of emotional information processing, and mind and consciousness would appear to be independent of brain and body. ...The DNA molecules have the information that makes the brain and body, and the bodymind seems to share the information. (pp. 35).

    Pert (1997) explains that the molecules of emotion run every system in the body, and this communication system is in effect a demonstration of the body-mind intelligence. This is an intelligence wise enough to seek wellness, and one that can potentially keep humans healthy and disease free without the modern high-tech medical intervention humans now rely on. Up to now, scientists thought of the brain and its extension the central nervous system, primarily as an electrical communication system. Receptors and their ligands have come to be seen as "information molecules" – the basic units of a language used by cells throughout the organism to communicate across systems such as the endocrine, neurological, gastrointestinal, and even the immune system.

    Pert states that the placebo effect, and the expectation of improvement actually changing outcome, is an extremely powerful demonstration of the involvement of the mind in healing. According to Pert negative emotions, such as fear, anger, anxiety, and negative stressors, cause glands such as the pituitary, endocrine, and adrenal glands to produce harmful chemicals such as dopamine, adrenaline, and cortisol that enter and weaken the cells. Positive emotions and exercises, such as prayer, meditation and laughter, result in the production of calming and healing chemicals such as melatonin and seratonin, to name a few. Up until the present, humans knew that "stress" was harmful, but now it can be explained exactly how it affects one physiologically (Pert, 1997).

For many years it was believed that the brain sent messages to the body. It was a one-way messaging system. Several years ago I had an elderly gentleman in a therapy session that was recovering from a stroke. At that point he had still had numbness and limited use of his arms and hands and feet (distal appendages). His doctor told him he would have to wait, probably a few more months, for new neural connections or passages in his brain to be created in order to stimulate the muscles and nerves to these areas. I explained muscle proprioceptors and the two-way muscle messaging system to him and said I wanted to experiment. It was ok with him, and I began doing intense focused work on these areas, thinking that the body could stimulate its need to the brain centers instead. We made remarkable progress in the next several weeks.

Coincidentally, about two months later I attended the National Institute for the Clinical Application of Behavioral Medicine (NICABM) Conference. The keynote speaker was Dr. Candace Pert. She spoke about the ground-breaking discovery and ability to prove the information network happening throughout out the body. The body sends messages to the brain, as well and vice versa. I was so excited, this was the first I heard of it, and I felt validated in my belief. I forced myself not to jump up and yell: "Yes, Yes, thank you. I just knew it!"

I have had similar sessions with a two other stroke patients at the clinic since then.

"The important thing is this: To be ready at any moment to sacrifice what you are for what you could become."
- *Charles Dubois*

Neurolinguistic Programming

Another treatment method is Neurolinguistic Programming (NLP). It is an approach to personal and professional excellence that combines concepts about communication, internal experience, the effects of language on humans, modeling excellent behavior, and how to use one's brain (Adler, 2002). McDermott and Jago (2002) describe how to use NLP in brief therapy. They focus on practical aspects, and present many case studies to illustrate not only that it works, but also how it worked for particular clients and issues.

Neurolinguistic Programming is a system that uses the language of the mind to achieve specific and desired outcomes consistently (Walter & Bayat, 2003). A person's nervous system experiences "the world around them through the five senses: visual, auditory, kinesthetic, olfactory, and gustatory. These experiences are coded, ordered, and sorted (programmed) as specific representations that can be replayed through language and other non-verbal forms of communication" (p. 163). NLP is a tool to help one to understand these programs and use them to meet their desired goals.

Walter and Bayat (2003) also express the need

to set a goal, to be positive, detailed, realistic, set criteria for success, and to be prepared to make personal sacrifices. They also point out the need to model one's own or a specific person's behavior by mastering three aspects that make up that behavior: the beliefs, the physiology, and the specific thought processes (strategies). "Success is more likely if one defines what one wants and then takes the appropriate action to bring about their desired goal. This concept can be applied throughout the health service, particularly in helping patients take charge of their health" (pp. 252-253). Individual goal setting is an important part of the self-management essential for managing chronic pain.

This is the purpose of a study conducted using psychosocial and cognitive treatment approaches conducted by Davis and White (2006). Participant's experience of living with persistent pain and perception of how well they were managing pain were measured pre and post-test and showed a nonsignificant increase.

Another study conducted by Hekmat, Staats and Staats (2006) using cognitive/behavioral approaches explored the effect of the visualization of spiritual fantasies on the experience of acute pain. Results indicated that spiritual fantasies significantly improved pain threshold, pain tolerance, and reduced pain intensity and pain anxiety. Spiritual fantasies also improved participants' mood and self-efficacy. Results also suggest that application of spiritual fantasies in therapeutic intervention programs for pain, pain-related anxiety, and distress management may have beneficial effects for patients.

Milstein (2008) explains that when cure eludes patients with devastating conditions, healing measures become of utmost importance. Forging a spiritual connection among any patient and his or her significant others can restore a sense of control, meaning, and the ability to cope, allowing patients and families undergoing catastrophic events to shift from a state of hopelessness to wholeness. Facilitating spiritual connections can help families cope with grief or despair. Healing and curing can coexist with the clinical setting. By using a 'healing space', a spiritual intervention can serve as an experiential basis to restore a sense of order and meaning for patients and their families, improving their ability to cope and to attain a sense of wholeness.

Studies designed to assess spiritual interventions are rarely pursued because spiritual aspects are not fully embraced as part of conventional medical "culture". Establishing the value of a spiritual intervention may further the likelihood of its inclusion earlier in care by more practitioners. Strong empirical support exists for the association between pain catastrophizing, pain severity, perceived disability, occupational impairment, greater emotional distress, and increased analgesic medication use in persons with chronic noncancer pain.

This is shown in a study on interventions to decrease pain catastrophizing (Evans & Townsend, 2006). The study supported the feasibility and effectiveness of a comprehensive rehabilitation program that incorporates a psychoeducational intervention to decrease pain catastrophizing and promote utilization of adaptive cognitive pain coping strategies.

Guided imagery is one component of cognitive behavioral therapy (CBT) that frequently is used. Imagery has been defined as a dynamic, psychophysiologic process in which a person imagines, and experiences, an internal reality in the absence of external stimuli. What makes imagery clinically relevant is that a person who uses imagery may experience an affective, behavioral or physiologic response without a real stimulus event. Thus, mental imagery may be used to alter one's physiologic process, mental state, self-image, performance, or behavior. Battino (2000) defines guided imagery as any internal work that you do that involves thoughts and has a positive effect on health. This can range from 'positive thinking' to elaborately structured processes involving relaxation, meditation, and body postures. The common denominator is thoughts, and their effect on body function. The important factor is to guide the client to enhance their own natural healing processes via paths and sensations that are unique to them.

The Harvard Women's Health Watch (2004, pp. 4-5) explains that cognitive behavioral therapy teaches patients that their thoughts influence how they feel and behave. Its goal is to help them learn how to turn unproductive thought patterns into helpful ones. This may include learning how to shift focus from what they cannot do anymore to activities they can still enjoy, or adjusting expectations to minimize disappointment.

During cognitive behavioral therapy, fibromyalgia sufferers also learn how to adapt daily activities to prevent flare-ups caused by doing too much or lethargy caused by doing too little. It may require more than one strategy, but they can get some pain relief and feel a lot better about life. Menzies, Gill Taylor, and Bourguignon (2006) state that many researchers have reported that CBT with guided imagery as one component produced significant improvements in functional status and/or self-efficacy and reductions in individuals' pain, emotional distress, and tender point measures.

However, recent reviews of treatments for persons with FM have reported that although complementary modalities such as CBTs may be helpful to patients with FM, these interventions have not been adequately evaluated for their incremental effect. Most studies to date have investigated guided imagery as a component of CBTs for FM.

According to Menzies et al. two studies

investigated guided imagery as the sole CBT intervention in persons with FM. The purpose of their study was to investigate the effects of guided imagery on pain perception, functional status, and self-efficacy in persons with FM.

The intervention for one of their studies consisted of three guided imagery (GI) audiotapes that were used by study participants in the GI group during a 6-week treatment period and a 4-week follow-up period, to elicit a relaxation and/or imagery 4 3 response in persons with FM. The guided imagery intervention was not effective in modulating any measures of pain in this study.

These results are consistent with suggestions by other researchers that the pain experience may or may not be satisfactorily ameliorated through any one-treatment modality, including cognitive behavioral strategies such as guided imagery. Individuals diagnosed with FM may have become so accustomed to chronic pain that guided imagery could not produce responses that might be observed in individuals unaccustomed to such pain.

The subjective, private nature of pain, and the subjective nature of FM symptoms in general confound efforts to assess why the guided imagery intervention did not decrease reported pain, yet significantly increased GI participants' functional status and sense of self-efficacy for managing pain.

In another study, Menzies, Gill Taylor and Bourguignon (2006) conducted a study to investigate the effects of a 6-week intervention of guided imagery on pain level, functional status, and self-efficacy in persons with fibromyalgia; and to explore the dose-response effect of imagery use on outcomes.

This study demonstrated the "effectiveness of guided imagery in improving functional status and a sense of self-efficacy for managing pain and other symptoms of FM. However, participants' reports of pain did not change" (pp. 23-30). Because persons with FM suffer a chronic disease with no known cure, they may believe that the pain and accompanying difficulties in function are uncontrollable. In persons diagnosed with FM, pain has been shown to be influenced by psychosocial factors, as well as by the individual's level of self-efficacy. Further, self-efficacy has been found to improve in persons with FM who received cognitive behavioral interventions for symptom management (Menzies et al. 2006).

McDermott and O'Connor (1996) state that the consumer revolution tempts humans to think individuals are consumers of health, but they are not, they are its creators – by what they do, how they think, and how they live. Their bodies take in and metabolize not only air and food, but also time and experience. How they use the above creates their health from moment to moment. Modern medicine takes an objective, dissociated view of health. NLP theorizes that one needs also to understand it from the inside. Health and illness are both subjective and objective experiences. Every person's experience and inner world are different.

Jahnke (1999) contends that if one has internally agreed to make choices that equate with joy, satisfaction, and trust, then a positive physiological response occurs throughout the body, particularly in the immune system. In the past this was called "positive thinking" or "mental healing."

Most experts in the field of mind-body medicine and healing agree that both meditation and prayer are forms of focused intention. Both produce relaxation and shifts in brain-wave frequency and body chemistry. A lot of recent research has supported the role of prayer in the healing process.

Jahnke further explains that when one triggers the healing system with self-applied health enhancement methods and then they also trigger the power of the belief system, the capacity for heightened human potential, and for recovery from disease is greatly magnified. From ancient time through the present, the most revered healers have known that the human being has a vital self-healing capacity that is profoundly influenced by faith and emotional harmony. Soon self-healing will become as common as aspirin and antibiotics have been in the past. Jahnke also maintains that the effect of humor is well documented. Research on placebos, remissions, and miracles reflects the healing influence of belief.

Faith, forgiving and surrender are also powerful mental and spiritual factors in self-healing, as well as group support, accountability, and testimonials. All of these help to neutralize negative emotions and self-sabotaging beliefs. Jahnke believes that being accountable for honesty, purposeful work, joyfulness, service, family time, and play is one of the most potent tools for improvement of health or personal performance, because it means one will do what they say they will do. It is identical to integrity.

Those who master accountability are literally reborn through their own labor. Biologically this rebirth produces a fantastic medicine within the human system. Together with health enhancement and self-healing methods, accountability is an astounding force. Accountability in relation to the self-healing methods produces vigilant practice, and vigilant practice makes miracles possible (Jahnke, 1999).

What makes psychosomatic treatment unique and effective? Sivik (2005) explains that if a person is indivisible and complete, physically, spiritually, psychosocially, and creatively, and if disease involve the whole person, then disease somehow expresses and is expressed by, and through, and thanks to, all aspects of human life. To help people restore or develop and improve their capacity to deal with life events and with their mortality, we need to approach the person simultaneously on all levels of consciousness: subconscious, preconscious,

conscious, and the awareness of consciousness.

I have observed that not all therapies are effective on everyone. A client who has fibromyalgia shared an experience that happened to her several years ago. She went to a practitioner for hypnotherapy using visualization. She went because she was tired of living with pain and had a perceived energy blockage. The therapist tried to do visualization with her, telling her to picture a black screen, like a movie screen, and then put images up there of what you want, or desired outcomes. She said that the screen continually stayed blank. She really wanted to help herself and find out what the problem was. The therapist said that she was one of the few people that he could not successfully put under hypnosis. She went for about 10 sessions, for 1 to 1 ½ hours a session.

He thought it was a control issue and she thinks not. It was either his technique or she was not really ready to let go, even though she believed that she was. She was able to go back in time; she could feel herself in different situations and in touch with different emotions. But she was completely unable to go forward in time, nor to make any projections. She is not sure if it was a belief system or resistance. Yet she was not aware of resisting on any level.

Although there have been some studies to the contrary, I believe that Psychoneuroimmunology and Neurolinguistic Programming can be effective bodymind processes, and that continued practice and research will be significant in this area. Also, research is showing that negative emotions result in negative or harmful chemicals being released into the body's cells, and positive emotions and beliefs result in beneficial and healing chemicals being released into the cells. Altering one's attitudes and beliefs can lead to a healthier physiology.

> *"Since almost all medications until recently were placebos, the history of medical treatment can be characterized largely as the history of the placebo effect."*
>
> — Arthur K. Shapiro

Placebo Response

The next area of examination is placebo response. The word "placebo" itself means, "I shall please" in Latin (Brody, 2000). It is a mysterious phenomenon of the mind working in tandem with the body to enhance healing. When a certain set of circumstances is present ill persons seem to improve greatly in what at first seems an inexplicable way. Placebo response occurs when one receives certain types of messages or signals from the environment around them. These messages work in some fashion to alter the meaning of their state of health or illness. The old thoughts one attributes to an illness might have been that it is "scary, I don't know what's causing it, or no one cares what happens to me." And the new thoughts may be "Now I know this is going to get better," or "people around me really seem concerned about my health."

Brody further explains that the placebo response is not restricted to symbols or signals that have no other possible impact on the body. A pill, injection, or surgical procedure, for instance, could easily have both a direct effect on the body by means understood by the usual biomedical theories, and also a symbolic impact which gives rise to a placebo response. He also explains that the human body is capable of producing many substances, which can heal a wide variety of illnesses, and make them feel generally healthier and more energized. When the body simply secretes these substances on its own, one has what is often termed "spontaneous healing."

Sometimes one's body is slow to react and a message from outside can serve as a wake-up call to their inner pharmacy. The placebo response can thus be seen as the reaction of the inner pharmacies to that wake-up call – the message of new meaning. Brody (2000) states that family physicians should be particularly interested in the placebo response. Bodily change can be negative as well as positive (nocebo effects). If we fail to understand the placebo response, we may unwittingly do harm. Because of the therapeutic usefulness of the placebo response and the way that it is intertwined with other elements of everyday practice it would seem that family practice investigators would be especially skilled at addressing the research difficulties. More attention should be paid to the placebo response and promoting a high priority to its research among primary care investigators and multidisciplinary research teams.

Signs are almost always given when one is facing illness or disease. But, according to Emery (2000) individuals must learn to look for and recognize these signs, taking appropriate action to recover their balance and restore or maintain their health. It is important to learn effective ways of connecting with the intuitive mind and receiving invaluable information and insights. Along the way an individual may have to change their physical regimen and old, unhealthy patterns of thought, emotion, and belief.

Access to one's inner physician increases an individual's ability in maintaining every facet of well-being, if one learns how to eradicate the thoughts, language patterns, beliefs, and actions that have limited their ability to stay healthy and happy in the past. An individual already has the power to think themselves well and to call on the tremendous healing resources within when confronting any major health challenge (Emery, 2000). "It inevitably disturbs pharmaceutical manufacturers that in most of their clinical trials the placebos, the 'fake' drugs, prove to be about as effective as their engineered chemical cocktails" (Greenberg, 2003, pp. 76-81).

Placebos are effective in treating diseases as well as depression. Brown (1998) has proposed placebo pills as the first treatment for patients with mild or moderate depression. Patients would be told that they are getting a remedy with no active ingredient, but that should not dampen the pill's effectiveness. Even knowing that, the placebo pills still worked.

The history of medicine is the history of the placebo, according to Benson (1997). He says that the reputation of physicians was built on and cultivated by the success of remembered wellness and on the three modes of belief inspired healing: the belief of an individual in a treatment, the belief of the caregiver, or their mutual beliefs. He observes that the Comanche Indians had intense faith in their tribal medicine men. A patient's imagination was often called upon in rituals that seemed to hasten recovery. Benson quotes Seneca, the Latin philosopher who lived from about 4 B.C. to A.D. 65, appreciated the role of hope, saying, "It is part of the cure to wish to be cured. For most of history, individuals bore responsibility for their own health" (p. 110).

Benson further explains that humans are at a turning point in the history of belief in healing, and for the spiritual quality of life. It has taken just over 150 years for humanity to come full circle – to abandon and then redeem the beliefs that aided the survival of men and women from the very start. He notes that Americans have trouble believing that rest, relief from stress and the indulgence of time can be healing. Doctors in Europe send patients to government-financed spas to relax and heal, a practice that is unheard of in the States. Benson, Corliss and Cowley (2004) state that placebos are just the beginning. And that studies suggest that any number of soothing emotional experiences can improve our physical health. Yoga, prayer or simple deep-breathing exercises can help counter the effects of chronic stress. The body produces more nitric oxide when deeply relaxed, and this molecule acts as an antidote to cortisol and other potentially toxic stress hormones.

Can we teach ourselves to be healthier? That is the central question of mind-body medicine. Stressful life circumstances are sometimes inescapable. Mind body techniques can improve almost anyone's quality of life. Mind-body medicine offers a starting place. If it fulfills half its promise, it could reduce medical costs while improving our health and our lives. Whatever its limitations, it has the advantage of doing no harm.

Barzini (1993) suggests that Americans are compelled to act because they believe the main purpose of a man's life is to solve problems, despite the fact that the body is the greatest problem-solver there is. It quietly and perpetually sustains life, overcoming billions of obstacles without conscious orders to do it, so individuals do not trust it. Their doctor's first impulse is to prescribe something for them. They fully expect to emerge from these visits with a prescription in hand.

Doctors are reluctant to admit that the placebo effect contributes to the success of the treatments they recommend or perform, according to Hofling (1955). Many years ago he said that the evidence shows that every specialty and treatment benefits from affirmative beliefs and remembered wellness, and that every treatment is equally vulnerable to the negative repercussions of the *nocebo* effect. "Nocebo is from the Latin 'I shall harm'. The nocebo effect is very important because it adds to the scientific evidence that expectancy can produce bodily changes" (pp. 103-107).

Another study, by Fawzy (1993) demonstrated

the value of self-care in potentially life-threatening causes of malignant melanoma. Patients received education on the disease itself, and on basic nutrition, stress management, and coping skills. They also received psychological support in a group setting and one-on-one with staff members, and were less apt to have the disease recur and less apt to die than patients who did not get this help.

Inui (1994) believes the days of doctors serving as mere diagnosticians and as prescribers of sophisticated drugs are numbered. He thinks doctors will be sought for their counsel and social wisdom, returning to their roots as healers. He recalls serving as a physician in a Native American population. He was asked by a Navajo in New Mexico what he did. He replied, "I give out pills." "Ah," the questioner said, "you are the low sort of medicine man. We have two sorts. The high sort, we go to for counseling and care" (pp. 89-90).

Shure wrote in 1965 about the concept of placebo surgery. She knew a surgeon who thought nothing of performing an oblique lower right quadrant incision, then suturing without entering the abdominal cavity in patients who had emotional problems manifested by pain in the abdomen. His results were excellent and as one might expect his operative mortality and morbidity were exceptionally low. Certainly this is not common, and she doubts whether anyone else would have done such procedures. However she is certain that thousands of appendectomies and hysterectomies are done yearly as placebos.

As a young doctor taking over a medical practice in a rural area, Vincent (1994) began by cleaning out the pill room. Feeling righteous, he marched out back and threw out the tall jar of coated, purple capsules labeled "placebo" he found on the shelf. But as his practice grew, he was surprised that a significant number of patients with a variety of medical conditions complained that his treatments were not working as well as the previous doctor's. He heard statements like: "the prescriptions you gave me didn't work as well as those purple pills Dr. Kass gave me, for my arthritis," and "do you have the purple pills for my blood pressure?" He soon got on the phone to the drug company and ordered a gallon jug. And because his patients believed in them, the placebos worked wonders. "There is no question that having to humble myself enough to use the purple pills made me a better doctor. In those days, I had a few things to learn about listening to and paying attention to patients. It is really the purpose of the person giving the purple pills that affect patients."

Two psychiatrists, Park and Covi (1965) conducted a study on truth-telling in the use of placebos. They enrolled 15 new patients diagnosed with neurosis in a trial and gave them a bottle of pills. They told the patients frankly that they were sugar pills, which contain no active medicine. They added that many patients had gotten better after taking one of the pills three times a day for a week. When 14 of the 15 subjects returned the new symptom checklists showed that 13 of the 14 had significantly reduced symptoms.

Park and Covi then actually held conversations with their subjects to ascertain what was going on inside their heads. They learned that the subjects could be divided into three groups. The first group took them at their word and assumed they were taking sugar pills. The second decided one could not trust psychiatry researchers and believed the pills were really some kind of tranquilizer. The third group was unsure of what they had received.

Park and Covi noted that the first two groups reported more substantial improvement then the uncertain group. And those convinced they were getting "real" drugs also reported a number of side effects they felt; but those thinking they had a placebo reported no side effects at all. The researchers then asked the "certain placebo" subjects how they could account for getting better. Half said they got better because they took the placebo, and the other half claimed they improved because somehow they had drawn upon their own innate abilities to cope. One woman reported that every time she took one of the placebos, she reminded herself that she really could do something to better her own condition. Other subjects testified they appreciated not getting an active drug and so they were spared the side effects and risk of addiction. Also, the "certain real drug" group saw their symptoms improving which reinforced their views that the pills were genuine medicine (Park & Covi, 1965).

    The top-down response of the brain quickly scans its existing inventory of behavior patterns to match the new information. It is most likely to be triggered in situations where the mind-body unit regards itself as being in danger. Brody (2000) contends that since illness is a threat to the organism, the brain may well have stored in its memory files certain pathways of healing. These signals can be sent to the inner pharmacy to stimulate the release of healing chemicals. "If a message is then received that resembles something that the person expects to be associated with healing, that might be enough to trigger one of the stored top-down reaction pathways, leading to a release from the inner pharmacy, followed by bodily healing" (pp. 65-66).

    Levine, Gordon and Fields (1978) conducted a study that involved giving placebo injections for wisdom tooth extractions. The study suggested that placebo pain relief may have been caused by the release of endorphins in the brain. The placebo is helping to redefine medicine and healing in terms that declare the power of self-healing resources.

    Jahnke (1999) studied testimonials that have not been in favor until recently. They were historically seen as unproveable. They dramatically support personal change. He has found that empirically, through working with individuals and groups, that there is a resident wisdom within each person. When incorrect information, reactive emotions, and false attitudes that spring from fear and guilt are polished away, the light of wisdom shines.

Sharing testimonials is the way in which this wisdom is communicated. Jahnke suggests cultivating the following formula: Cultivate the influence of positive emotions, such as joy and gratitude. Cultivate the influence of faith – faith in the "mystery," faith in science, and faith in what one has discovered one's self. Cultivate humor and fun. Neutralize anxiety, frustration, and fear. Seek the support of others, and serve others by supporting them. Listen for the stories and testimonials that confirm inner potential to reach preferred conditions and circumstances.

It appears that testimonials and "soft" studies are gaining approval and credence. The "stories" of people in remission prove that self-healing is an undeniable and obtainable promise. Hearing the stories of others regarding their experiences with the self-healing methods or their breakthroughs in seeking emotional balance or their breakthroughs in faith can assist others in their search to improve their health (Jahnke, 1999).

Langer (1990) maintains the placebo effects are real and powerful. Who is doing the healing when one takes a placebo? Why can't an individual just say, "repair this ailing body?" Why must we fool our minds in order to enlist our own powers of self-healing? Using placebos, hypnosis, autosuggestion, faith healing, visualization, and positive thinking, one controls their health, or the course of their disease without really knowing that they do. Now may be the time to learn how to recognize and use one's control over illness. Humans should be able to "take" a placebo instead of a pill. Conceiving of the mind and body as one means that wherever an individual puts the mind, they may be able to put their bodies. The mind may have to be fooled to reach a healthy place.

Once humans learn how to put it there consciously, the evidence suggests that the body may well follow. Crum and Langer (2007) also state that the placebo effect is any effect that is not attributed to an actual pharmaceutical drug or remedy, but is attributed to the individual's mind-set. The therapeutic benefit of the placebo effect is so widely accepted that accounting for it has become a standard in clinical drug trials. This is to distinguish pharmaceutical effects from the placebo effect and the placebo effect from other possible confounding factors, including spontaneous remission and the natural history of the condition.

Battino (2007) explains that expectation is central to the power of the placebo effect. There are literally thousands of papers on this subject and many good books. Double-blind studies are done on new pharmaceuticals and treatments to separate the effect of the active agent from that of a placebo. With respect to pain management it is well known that placebos are about 55% as effective as the medication, and placebo injections are more effective than placebo pills.

Siegel (1996) reveals that the placebo effect can change the body chemistry, and change the internal hormones. It shows that mind and body are a single unit. If you read a chemotherapy protocol with all of its side effects to a patient, and then inject him with saline (no medicine), the patient's hair falls out! According to Brody (2000), even if we cannot control or guarantee the placebo response, the possibility remains that we can harness it to heal faster, stay healthier and generally function better. Along with the concept of the inner pharmacy, it is the most important new concept. I'm proposing that, if we line up the scientific clues in the right order, we will master a variety of means by which we can employ the placebo response and the inner pharmacy to benefit ourselves.

Jahnke (1999) states that when people learn about the healer within themselves and then take action to care for their own physical, mental, emotional, and spiritual health, they are transformed. Victims of life's problems become independent and empowered creators of better health, greater joy, and positive living. Instead of handing over the power to others, they retain the authority to make their own choices and to participate in an exciting era of change.

Juhan (1987) explains that the relationship between our experiences, our feelings, and our body chemistry are undoubtedly far more intricate than we can presently imagine. We have seen how specific mental states effect specific glandular secretions, circulatory patterns, and organ functions. If we now remind ourselves that every nerve cell is itself a type of gland, a gland whose chemical secretions are the mechanisms for carrying action potentials from cell to cell, we can appreciate the fact that there is probably no limit to the influencing of function and behavior by feelings and attitudes.

Learning to be sick involves one's own physiological and emotional responses to certain stimuli one does not like, responses that either reinforce or add their own flavor headache. Or they can be chronic and devastating, such as the long-term withering of mental and physical vitality due the constant and unresolved stress. Have I learned to deal with stress by minimizing my losses, recuperate efficiently, and move on? Or, have I learned to ignore unpleasant symptoms until the damage is so extensive that I am forced to succumb? Or, have I learned to react to symptoms with additional diverting symptoms, discomforts of my own making, which may effectively mask the original problem, but which can join it in a vicious circle that can make its consequences far more severe (Juhan, 1987)?

Each of these vicious circles requires a *feeling* or an *attitude* just as much as it needs a chemical change to perpetuate itself. In the absence of negative emotions, many destructive processes are unable to continue. There is no depression, no drop in brain norepinephrine; no anxiety, no rise in lactate levels in the blood; no helplessness, no gastric ulcers. This highly correlated relationship between certain feeling states and certain physiological functions may seem like a riddle or even like nonsense, if one does not recognize that humans are to a large degree learning to cultivate various states of health and disease, just like they learned to walk or to read.

Humans also continue to discover that this miracle, the body, can be one's greatest enemy. It often reacts in ways that appear capricious, unconscious, and cruel. The same laws and elements that govern it may also sicken and even destroy it with no compunctions. The very cells and systems that are designed to sustain and protect humans can turn viciously against them and wreak havoc with their existence.

Juhan continues to explain that by the time the discomfort we are suffering becomes greater than the discomfort of changing our ways, the physical damage has already been done. It is this extreme psychological ambiguity of discomfort and pain itself that diverts us from the real causes of limitations and from the practical steps we could be taking to move beyond them. If feeling states, attitudes, behavioral, and physiological habits can start large circles of inter-related processes turning in vicious directions, might not different states, attitudes, and habits start turning in healthy ones? And can we not learn new ones?

Juhan states that once humans have lost sight of these continual and life-long changes that are occurring in all of their tissues and in their over-all patterns of coordinated behavior, they inevitably lose sight of another most significant fact. They are personally responsible for the tendencies of those changes and for the results they create in their lives. By refusing to consciously confront issues and consequences, they only narrow their range of possible choices; by ignoring their options they make certain choices by default; and by passively accepting the notion that they have no real choices to make, perhaps they make the most irrevocable choice of all.

The body is an object that inescapably conditions one's perceptions, thoughts, and feeling, which, in turn, condition every cell, every organ, and every function of physiology, for better or for worse. Awareness and the will to participate actively in one's own development are personal action principles. One must open oneself up to the messages the body is sending. They must consciously seek out the information that will clarify and complete the body image; and mentally and physically engage themselves in the internal events that awareness reveals if they are to have any hope of positively affecting their course (Juhan, 1987).

Lipton (2005) states that when the mind is engaged in negative suggestions that can damage health, the negative effects are referred to as the nocebo effect. It can be as powerful as the placebo effect. By their words and their demeanor, physicians can convey hope-deflating messages to their patients.

Nocebo cases suggest that physicians, parents, and teachers can remove hope by programming one to believe one is powerless. Lipton suggests that an individual can filter their life with rose-colored beliefs that will help their body grow or they can use a dark filter that turns everything black and makes their body/mind more susceptible to disease. One can live a life of fear or live a life of love. If one chooses to see a world full of love, their body will respond by growing in health. If one chooses to believe that they live in a dark world full of fear, their body's health will be compromised as they physiologically close themselves down in a protection response. Rose-colored glasses are necessary for one's cells to thrive.

Lipton explains that the conscious mind is the "self," the voice of one's own thoughts. While one focuses on those thoughts, the subconscious mind is going to manage their affairs the way it was programmed. One's behaviors may not be of their own creation because most of their fundamental behaviors were downloaded without question from observing other people. The learned behaviors and beliefs acquired from other people may not support the goals of one's conscious mind.

The biggest impediments to realizing the successes of which one dreams are the limitations programmed into the subconscious. These limitations influence their behavior, and play a major role in determining their physiology and health. They try repeatedly to override the subconscious program, but it is usually met with resistance because the cells are obligated to adhere to the program (Lipton, 2005).

According to Hoffman, Harrington and Fields (2005) the extent to which administration of placebo treatments can result in real and clinically significant changes has been subject to both hype and controversy, but more has been learned about this phenomenon than is widely realized. Particularly in the area of pain and analgesia, impressive strides have been made in describing the magnitude, probability of occurrence, and potency of responses to placebos. Also in understanding the underlying psychological and neural mechanism that mediate placebo analgesic responses.

What is the placebo worth? Spiegel (2008) suggests that "the doctor-patient relationship is a crucial part of the placebo's value. A good doctor-patient relationship can tangibly improve patient's responses to treatment, regardless of whether a placebo is involved" (p. 967).

I believe that the research indicates that placebos can be as or more effective than medications in individual situations. Also, given the choice, many patients would prefer not to risk the side effects or chemical reactions to medicines. Furthermore, because there are no healing properties in a placebo, the healing most likely is coming from within the patient.

"How common illness is, how tremendous the spiritual change that it brings."
— *Mike Denney*

Chapter 4. Fibromyalgia: Symptoms and Beliefs

Fibromyalgia is an elusive illness. Millions of Americans are affected by fibromyalgia, a mysterious debilitating disorder. Here's what is known so far about its symptoms, causes, and risk factors. It is a widely misunderstood and sometimes misdiagnosed chronic condition, commonly characterized by widespread muscle pain, fatigue, concentration issues, and sleep problems. According to the National Fibromyalgia Association, it affects an estimated 10 million people, mainly women, in the United States alone. The severity of fibromyalgia symptoms can vary from one person to the next and may fluctuate even in a single individual, depending on such factors as time of day or the weather. Because it is a chronic condition, in most cases fibromyalgia symptoms never disappear entirely. The good news is that fibromyalgia isn't progressive or life threatening, and treatments can help alleviate many symptoms.

Fibromyalgia: The Symptoms

The symptoms of fibromyalgia and their severity vary widely, although pain and fatigue are nearly always present. Major symptoms of fibromyalgia include:

- **Pain.** Some fibromyalgia patients report discomfort in one or more specific areas of their body, while others may experience overall pain in their muscles, ligaments, and tendons. Certain areas, such as the back of the head, upper back and neck, elbows, hips, and knees may be particularly sensitive to touch or pressure and are described clinically as tender points. The degree and type of pain can range from aching, tenderness, and throbbing to sharper shooting and stabbing sensations. Intense burning, numbness, and tingling may also be present.

- **Fatigue.** If you've ever been knocked off your feet by a bad case of the flu, you have a general idea of how tired some people with fibromyalgia can feel. Though some fibromyalgia patients experience only mild fatigue, many report feeling completely drained of energy, both physically and mentally, to the point that exhaustion interferes with all daily activities.

- **Memory problems.** Difficulty concentrating and remembering are common cognitive symptoms in people with fibromyalgia.

- **Sleep disturbances.** Research has shown that the deepest stages of sleep in patients with fibromyalgia are constantly interrupted by bursts of brain activity, causing feelings of exhaustion even after a seemingly good night's rest. Other problems such as sleep apnea, restless legs syndrome, and teeth grinding (bruxism) are also common among fibromyalgia sufferers.

- **Irritable bowel syndrome (IBS).** Symptoms of IBS, including diarrhea, constipation, abdominal pain, and bloating, are present in many people with fibromyalgia.

Other common symptoms
- Headaches, migraines, and facial pain
- Depression, anxiety, or mood changes
- Painful menstrual periods
- Dizziness
- Dry mouth, eyes, and skin
- Heightened sensitivity to noise, odors, bright lights, and touch

Symptom Triggers
The following factors can worsen the symptoms of fibromyalgia:
- Changes in weather (too cold or too humid)
- Too much or too little exercise
- Too much or too little rest
- Stress and anxiety
- Depression

Some patients also report that pain and stiffness are worse in the morning.

Causes of Fibromyalgia
While the exact cause of fibromyalgia remains a mystery, doctors do know that patients with the disorder experience an increased sensation of pain due to a glitch in the central nervous system's processing of pain information. Studies have shown that people with fibromyalgia also have certain

physiological abnormalities, such as elevated levels of certain chemicals called nuerotransmitters that help transmit pain signals (thus amplifying, or "turning up," the signals in the brain's pain-processing areas). In some cases, an injury or trauma, especially to the cervical spine, or a bacterial or viral illness, may precede a diagnosis of fibromyalgia. This has caused researchers to speculate that infections may be triggers as well.

Fibromyalgia Risk Factors

A number of factors can increase the odds that you may develop fibromyalgia. These include:

- **Gender.** Fibromyalgia is more common among women than men.

- **Age.** Symptoms usually appear during middle age, but can also manifest in children and older adults.

- **History of rheumatic disease.** People who have been diagnosed with a rheumatic disorder — chronic inflammatory conditions — such as rheumatoid arthritis and lupus are at increased risk of also developing fibromyalgia.

- **Family history.** Having a relative who suffers from fibromyalgia puts you at increased risk.

- **Sleep problems.** Doctors aren't sure whether sleep disturbances are a cause or a symptom of fibromyalgia — but sleep disorders, including restless legs syndrome and sleep apnea have been cited as possible fibromyalgia triggers.

I believe that fibromyalgia is a puzzling

syndrome. It is difficult to diagnose, and difficult to treat. Each fibromyalgia patient is unique in his or her symptoms and in the types of treatments to which they respond. Also there are conflicting theories of what fibromyalgia is, and its causes.

The National Institute of Arthritis and Musculoskeletal and Skin Diseases Department (NIAMS) of the National Institutes of Health (2004) describes and explains fibromyalgia syndrome as a common and chronic disorder, characterized by widespread muscle pain, fatigue, and multiple tender points. These points are specific places on the body – on the neck, shoulders, back, hips, and upper and lower extremities – where people with fibromyalgia feel pain in response to slight pressure. In addition they may experience sleep disorders, morning stiffness, headaches, irritable bowel syndrome, painful menstrual periods, numbness or tingling of the extremities, restless legs syndrome, temperature sensitivity, cognitive and memory problems (sometimes referred to as "fibro fog"), or a variety of other symptoms.

"Unlike a disease, which is a medical condition with a specific cause or causes and recognizable signs and symptoms, a syndrome is a collection of signs, symptoms and medical problems that tend to occur together but are not related to a specific, identifiable cause" (p. 2).

NIAMS states that fibromyalgia affects 3 to 6 million – or as many as one in 50 – Americans. For unknown reasons, between 80 and 90 percent of those diagnosed with fibromyalgia are women; however, men and children also can be affected. Most people are diagnosed during middle age, although the symptoms often become present earlier in life.

They further explain that the causes of fibromyalgia are unknown, but there are probably a number of factors involved. Many people associate the development of fibromyalgia with a physically or emotionally stressful or traumatic event. Researchers are examining other causes, including problems with how the central nervous system (the brain and spinal cord) processes pain.

Some scientists speculate that a person's genes may regulate the way his or her body processes painful stimuli. According to this theory, people with fibromyalgia may have a gene or genes that cause them to react strongly to stimuli that most people would not perceive as painful. However, those genes – if they, in fact, exist - have not been identified (pp. 3-4).

According to NIAMS fibromyalgia is diagnosed based on two criteria. The presence of tender points and widespread pain that affects all four quadrants of the body lasting more than 3 months. Pain is considered to be widespread when it affects all four quadrants of the body; that is, you must have pain in both your right and left sides as well as above and below the waist to be diagnosed with fibromyalgia.

The American College of Rheumatology also has designated 18 sites on the body as possible tender points. For fibromyalgia diagnosis, a person must have 11 or more tender points. One of these predesignated sites is considered a true tender point only if the person feels pain upon the application of 4 kilograms of pressure to the site. People who have fibromyalgia certainly may feel pain at other sites, too, but those 18 standard possible sites on the body are the criteria used for classification (NIAMS, 2004).

A fibromyalgia tender point is unlike a trigger point that is tender when compressed and may give rise to referred pain and tenderness elsewhere on the body (Starlanyl & Copeland, 2000). However, according to Long (2004) fibromyalgia is a syndrome, a set of symptoms and findings commonly occurring together, and has not been officially assigned a disease state. Many physicians do not understand the diagnosis or its treatment or may be unwilling to make the diagnosis. Also, many physicians do not understand the cause, and confuse cause and effect. That is, they often blame the discomfort of a minor trauma for causing depression rather than assigning blame for exaggerated pain response to fibromyalgia with concomitant depression (Long, 2004).

Fibromyalgia is the commonest cause of widespread pain (Bennett, 1995), yet it may remain undiagnosed for a long time. The word is derived from the Greek, *algia* meaning pain; *myo* indicating muscle; *fibro* meaning connective tissue of tendons and ligaments. *Syndrome* means a group of signs and symptoms that occur together and that characterize a particular abnormality. For many years the medical profession called it by many names, including "chronic rheumatism" and "fibrositis" (pp. 269-275).

If there is a physically traumatic initiating event, these changes in the way the central nervous system processes pain seem to worsen. A patient may be sensitive to odors, sounds, lights, and vibrations that others do not even notice. Also, sleep disturbances, a swollen feeling, and exercise intolerance are significantly related.

Simons, Travell, and Simons (1999) state that it is now firmly established that a central nervous system (CNS) dysfunction is primarily responsible for the increased pain sensitivity of FMS. FM is not a musculoskeletal disorder. It should be called 'Central Nervous System-myalgia', that is where the dysfunction is located, not in the fibers of your muscles, although there may be cellular changes caused by the biochemical FMS dysfunction. FM is a biochemical disorder, and these biochemicals affect the whole body.

Wolfe et al. (1997) state that it is not progressive. If it becomes worse over time, then there is some perpetuating or aggravating factor or some coexisting condition that has not been addressed. If you identify that factor and deal with it thoroughly and promptly, your symptoms should ease considerably. According to Gerwin (1999) FM is not a catchall, wastebasket diagnosis. It is not a disease with a known cause and well-understood mechanisms for producing symptoms. "A syndrome is a specific set of signs and symptoms that occur together. FM is not the same as chronic myofascial pain (CMP), because there is not such a thing as a fibromyalgia trigger point. Trigger points are part of myofascial pain, not FMS" (pp. 209-215).

(Wittrup, Wiik, & Danneskild-Samsoe, 1999, pp. 273-277). Bennett and Jacobsen (1994) state "Initiating events often activate biochemical changes, causing a cascade of symptoms. Unremitting grief, cumulative trauma, protracted labor, open-heart surgery, and even inguinal hernia repair have all been initiating events for FMS" (pp. 721-746).

Ingerman (1991) says that physical illness can also be believed as a symptom of soul loss. For shamans the world over, illness has always been seen as a spiritual predicament: a loss of soul or a diminishment of essential spiritual energy. Often when one gives away their power they become ill.

Because the universe cannot stand a void, if they are missing pieces of themselves, an illness might fill in that place. Soul retrieval is for everyone who wants to open his or her connection to self, to loved ones, to the earth. Contemporary psychology recognizes that parts of the self can become separated, leaving the individual estranged from his or her essential self. Many current therapies understand that if trauma is too severe, parts of the vital, feeling self will split off to lessen the impact of the trauma. Whenever "energy" gets "stuck", it creates illness.

Ingerman explains that if the soul has fled and the ego is stuck at the traumatic time, the being is no longer in harmony, and there is illness. Whether physical, or emotional, or spiritual illness, the being will manifest some problem at being stuck. Depression results when energy stops moving. Often you are able to change a problematic state of consciousness by physically moving your body so your energy starts flowing again.

Staranyl (2000) says that the first thing to do is form a recovery plan. Get a complete physical examination, and plan a course of treatment with the primary health provider. The treatment plan may include the use of medications, counseling, and referral to a psychologist or other kinds of lifestyle changes.

There are several areas in everyone's life amenable to positive changes. This includes what kinds of food are eaten, the amount of exposure to bright light, the amount of exercise, how restorative sleep is, how comfortable living quarters are, and the mind and spirit. Knowing how to change negative thought patterns into positive ones and how to harness the power of positive affirmations can help turn back depression and allow the self to live a richer, happier life in spite of having FMS (p. 9).

Starlanyl (1998) also says it is important to establish a medical team which could consist of a primary physician, a physiatrist, a bodywork therapist, and psychological support. Also, attend a support group for people with FMS. These people often become the very best supporters" (p. 35).

Control is a major causal determinant of health in both mind and body according to Pelletier (1994). There are many terms both in professional and public literature that are used to describe this aspect of personal control, including the *will to live, self-efficacy, internal locus of control, learned optimism, and empowerment.* There is substantial research underlying each of these terms, but there is a tremendous amount of overlap, and control clearly covers the common ground. A vital mind-body model describes a dynamic interaction between internal and external stressors and a person's internal and external responses to them according to Pelletier. Whether the challenge is inside or outside, it triggers a major positive or negative interaction between the mind and body. Which is first is often impossible to determine; nevertheless, this interaction is a major, in some cases the exclusive, determinant of a person's health or illness.

Through research therapeutic strategies have been developed to elicit and sustain a person's ability to buffer or eliminate the detrimental effects of stressors on the mind-body system. Healing means more than just physical healing. Pain may appear to be in the body, but in reality it is in consciousness. The areas of sensation are in the brain and throughout the neurological system, and then there is the communication of pain and hurt. The feeling one feels is the result of a complex process and is primarily the result of consciousness. As one works with consciousness, that will change the world of experience.

Pelletier (2002) also reports that currently the diseases that are killing more people in developed nations are not infectious; they are chronic, degenerative diseases. These diseases are inextricably related to psychological, lifestyle, environmental, social, and even spiritual factors.

Mind-body medicine is supported by the greatest body of scientific evidence, for the greatest number of conditions, and for the largest number of people. It has also gained the widest acceptance within the conventional healthcare system. Essential to all complementary and alternative medicine therapies is the point that the intervention or cure does not exist "outside" the individual, independent of "inside" changes in attitude, lifestyle, and orientation toward self and environment. Such an approach demands internal, psychological transformation and the active, ongoing involvement of the individual.

Over 80% of all medical symptoms are self-diagnosed, self-treated, and self-limiting without medical care. Healing is not always synonymous with complete cessation of all physical symptoms. Healing literally means "to make whole". From this perspective, illness can be viewed as an opportunity to reclaim wholeness and completeness, even in the face of ongoing disease. This can occur, however, only when the mind and body are integrated into a whole, healing force. (pp. 14-15)

Healing is a much larger action and it means learning to take charge of one's environment. (Grayson, 1997) It is healing the whole organism, the entire action of your being and life. In spiritual healing the process is automatic once you have clarified your consciousness, removed blockages, and recognized your connection to the infinite Mind of the universe.

Techniques such as visualization, affirmation, and holding good thoughts involve acts of willpower, which take place on the human level instead of at the higher level of spiritual realization that results in healing. However, although I am aware of contrary participants' accounts, there is research showing ineffective treatments aimed at the muscles.

During the past decade, scientific research has provided new insight into the development from an acute, localized musculoskeletal disorder towards chronic widespread pain/fibromyalgia according to Nijs and Van Houdenhove (2007). Their in-depth review of basic and clinical research explained that:

Fibromyalgia is characterized by sensitization of central pain pathways, and ongoing source of pain is required before the process of peripheral sensitization can establish central sensitizations. There is evidence that a stress response system dysfunction may play a role in central sensitization.

Moreover, inappropriate cognitions, emotions and behaviors may have a negative impact on the descending pain-inhibitory mechanisms. In order to prevent chronicity in acute or subacute musculoskeletal disorders, it seems crucial to limit the time course of afferent stimulation of peripheral nociceptors.

It is suggested the manual therapy might have the capacity to prevent chronicity. Exercise interventions should take the process of central sensitization into account by using low to moderate intensity. Also stress management techniques such as relaxation and breathing exercises may be useful in some cases (pp. 1-10).

The pathophysiology of fibromyalgia is unclear (Chakrabarty & Zoorob, 2007). Fibromyalgia clusters in families, suggesting a genetic predisposition. Environmental and psychological factors, which could impact various members of the same family, may contribute to the symptomatology of the disease. "Current theories of pathogenesis include central sensitization and hypothalamic-pituitary-adrenal axis dysregulation; however, more research is needed to determine a definite pathophysiology" (pp. 247-248). He states that the American Medical Association recognized Fibromyalgia Syndrome (FMS) as a true illness and a major cause of disability in 1987.

It is not curable right now, but it is very treatable, and there are quite a few ways in which patients can improve their health and quality of life considerably. Research supports FMS as a distinct clinical syndrome deserving of informed medical care and continued research to better understand chronic widespread pain. (Russell, 1999) The American College of Rheumatology, the American Medical Association, the World Health Organization, and the National Institutes of Health have all accepted FMS as a legitimate clinical entity.

FMS is a complex syndrome characterized by pain amplification, musculoskeletal discomfort, and systemic symptoms, according to Morris, Cruwys and Kidd (1998). They explain that in FMS, there is a generalized disturbance of the way in which pain is processed by the body. One definition is as a widespread allodynia and hyperalgesia. Allodynia means ordinary nonpainful sensations are experienced as pain sensations. Hyperalgesia means pain sensations are intensified and amplified. If there is a physically traumatic initiating event, these changes in the way the central nervous system processes pain seem to worsen. A patient may be sensitive to odors, sounds, lights, and vibrations that others do not even notice. Also, sleep disturbances, a swollen feeling, and exercise intolerance are significantly related.

The results of a study conducted by Hamilton et al. (2008) showed that sleep duration and quality were related to affect and fatigue, and the effects of inadequate sleep on negative affect were cumulative. In addition, an inadequate amount of sleep prevented affective recovery from days with a high number of negative events. The results lend support to the hypothesis that sleep is a component of allostatic load and has an upstream role in daily functioning, and that sleep should be a primary intervention target for people with FM.

Also, it not the same as Chronic Fatigue Immune Dysfunction Syndrome (CFIDS), "although they may be part of the same family of central nervous system dysfunction. FM is not an autoimmune condition, a mental illness, nor is it infectious" (Wittrup, Wiik, & Danneskild-Samsoe, 1999, pp. 273-277). Bennett and Jacobsen (1994) state "Initiating events often activate biochemical changes, causing a cascade of symptoms. Unremitting grief, cumulative trauma, protracted labor, open-heart surgery, and even inguinal hernia repair have all been initiating events for FMS" (pp. 721-746).

Fibromyalgia has been established as a complex syndrome. Starlanyl (1998) explains that FM seems to be the result of many neurotransmitter cascades. The neurotransmitter cascade can cause changes throughout the body, and many of these changes may start cascades of their own. Once these cascades get moving, a combination of peripheral and central factors join in to make the changes chronic, and the result is what we call FM. Every patient may have different neurotransmitters and other biochemical "informational substances" disrupted in different ways.

Informational substance is a relatively new, broad term that includes peptides, neurotransmitters, neuromodulators, growth factors, hormones, interleukins, cytokines, and similar substances. These are the biochemicals in the body that convey information from one part to another. Each information substance may be used in many different ways in the body and brain, and may affect many other information substances. One could think of oneself as a vast network of messages traveling in these dimensions at all times, even when asleep (Starlanyl, 1998).

Myofascial pain is probably the most common cause of musculoskeletal pain and small changes in the myofascia can cause great stress to other parts of the body (Imamura et al. 1997). In FM and chronic myofascial pain (CMP) the superficial fascia is often stuck. A patient may have FMS and CMP, and each condition requires separate attention.

Treatment must proceed carefully, as CMP needs to be treated locally, and its perpetuating factors need to be addressed. FM needs to be treated systemically, and its perpetuating factors need to be addressed. In a study of 96 patients, Gerwin (1995) found that 74% of the patients had only myofascial pain. 35% of the myofascial pain patients had generalized trigger point pain in three of four quadrants. These patients had CMP and not FMS, yet they had widespread pain. They had the symptoms of CMP, but not the generalized hypersensitivity and tender points of FMS. (As stated previously, a site is considered a tender point if the person feels pain upon the application of 4 kilograms of pressure to the site. Unlike a trigger point that is tender that when compressed may give rise to referred pain and tenderness elsewhere on the body.)

    Among the FMS patients in this study, 28% had only FMS. Among the FMS patients, 72% had both FMS and CMP. If you have both of these conditions (Gerwin, 1999) their coexistence will have a direct impact on every phase of your treatment. "FM is a chronic illness that can be controlled. Chronic myofascial pain is a condition that is potentially curable, unless there is a fixed, uncorrectable underlying cause. The focus of treatment for both conditions is to restore more normal functioning with minimized pain" (pp. 209-215).

    If you are living with constant pain, sometimes unbearable, that limits many of your former activities you have sufficient cause to be depressed. When neurotransmitter dysfunction, which is understood to be the cause of depression, is added you have a prescription for disaster (Starlanyl, 2000).

    The American Pain Society emphasizes a broad-based approach that combines pharmacologic and nonpharmacologic modalities for a condition with manifestations that are multiple and diffuse according to Sherman (2007). Educating the patient and encouraging the patient to become actively involved in treatment form the cornerstone of fibromyalgia syndrome management.

    Primary care physicians can usually provide continuing treatment in a regimen that typically includes pharmacotherapy for specific symptoms, as well as nonmedicinal treatments with an emphasis on exercise and cognitive-behavioral therapy strategies.

Ingerman (1991) says that physical illness can also be believed as a symptom of soul loss. For shamans the world over, illness has always been seen as a spiritual predicament: a loss of soul or a diminishment of essential spiritual energy. Often when one gives away their power they become ill. Because the universe cannot stand a void, if they are missing pieces of themselves, an illness might fill in that place. Soul retrieval is for everyone who wants to open his or her connection to self, to loved ones, to the earth.

Contemporary psychology recognizes that parts of the self can become separated, leaving the individual estranged from his or her essential self. Many current therapies understand that if trauma is too severe, parts of the vital, feeling self will split off to lessen the impact of the trauma. Whenever "energy" gets "stuck", it creates illness. Ingerman explains that if the soul has fled and the ego is stuck at the traumatic time, the being is no longer in harmony, and there is illness. Whether physical, or emotional, or spiritual illness, the being will manifest some problem at being stuck. Depression results when energy stops moving. Often you are able to change a problematic state of consciousness by physically moving your body so your energy starts flowing again.

Thorsen (1999) states that "Patients are disturbed that their family, friends and employers are placing demands on their bodies that can't be met. Lack of understanding about the neurophysiology of chronic pain syndromes and the advent of evidence-based medicine has often resulted in insufficient care for patients who need help" (pp. 463-467). Staranyl (2000) says that the first thing to do is form a recovery plan. Get a complete physical examination, and plan a course of treatment with the primary health provider. Starlanyl (1998) also says it is important to establish a medical team which could consist of a primary physician, a physiatrist, a bodywork therapist, and psychological support. It is important to make sure they are educated about the cognitive aspects of FMS. Sharing communications is one way to get care providers to work as a team. Write a letter of intent and make copies for each member of the team. List all members, and explain the part that each one plays. Include the pharmacist, dentist, spiritual advisor, etc. And let each know that you would like a copy of all reports sent to each other, as well as you.

Goldberg, Kerns and Rosenberg (1993) stress that a strong support system is essential to the quality of life. They suggest finding at least five reliable friends and family members who can be called upon when support is needed. Describe to them what you are experiencing, and educate them about FMS. "You may want them to go to health care appointments with you for a better understanding of FMS, what you need, and how they can be helpful. Also, attend a support group for people with FMS. These people often become the very best supporters" (p. 35).

Control is a major causal determinant of health in both mind and body according to Pelletier (1994). There are many terms both in professional and public literature that are used to describe this aspect of personal control, including the *will to live, self-efficacy, internal locus of control, learned optimism, and empowerment.*

There is substantial research underlying each of these terms, but there is a tremendous amount of overlap, and control clearly covers the common ground. A vital mind-body model describes a dynamic interaction between internal and external stressors and a person's internal and external responses to them according to Pelletier. Whether the challenge is inside or outside, it triggers a major positive or negative interaction between the mind and body. Which is first is often impossible to determine;

nevertheless, this interaction is a major, in some cases the exclusive, determinant of a person's health or illness. Through research therapeutic strategies have been developed to elicit and sustain a person's ability to buffer or eliminate the detrimental effects of stressors on the mind-body

However, the research presented herein indicates overall that the various hypnotic modalities are productive tools that should system. Healing means more than just physical healing. Pain may appear to be in the body, but in reality it is in consciousness. The areas of sensation are in the brain and throughout the neurological system, and then there is the communication of pain and hurt.

The feeling one feels is the result of a complex process and is primarily the result of consciousness. As one works with consciousness, that will change the world of experience. Pelletier (2002) also reports that currently the diseases that are killing more people in developed nations are not infectious; they are chronic, degenerative diseases. These diseases are inextricably related to psychological, lifestyle, environmental, social, and even spiritual factors.

Mindbody medicine is supported by the greatest body of scientific evidence, for the greatest number of conditions, and for the largest number of people. It has also gained the widest acceptance within the conventional healthcare system. Essential to all complementary and alternative medicine therapies is the point that the intervention or cure does not exist "outside" the individual, independent of "inside" changes in attitude, lifestyle, and orientation toward self and environment. Such an approach demands internal, psychological transformation and the active, ongoing involvement of the individual. Over 80% of all medical symptoms are self-diagnosed, self-treated, and self-limiting without medical care. Healing is not always synonymous with complete cessation of all physical symptoms. Healing literally means "to make whole". From this perspective, illness can be viewed as an opportunity to reclaim wholeness and completeness, even in the face of ongoing disease. This can occur, however, only when the mind and body are integrated into a whole, healing force. (pp. 14-15)

    Healing is a much larger action and it means learning to take charge of one's environment. (Grayson, 1997) It is healing the whole organism, the entire action of your being and life. In spiritual healing the process is automatic once you have clarified your consciousness, removed blockages, and recognized your connection to the infinite Mind of the universe. Techniques such as visualization, affirmation, and holding good thoughts involve acts of willpower, which take place on the human level instead of at the higher level of spiritual realization that results in healing.

    However, although I am aware of contrary participants' accounts, there is research showing ineffective treatments aimed at the muscles. Long's research (2004) states that modalities including massage, passive physical therapy treatments, chiropractic and acupuncture may feel good but do not actually provide any long-term medical benefit according to Holdcraft, Asefi, and Buchwald. (2003)

    Long also says that attempted treatment of individual symptoms usually leads to a never-ending search for the ideal treatment and a never-ending succession of futile therapeutic efforts. And Long explains that research by King et al. (2002) suggests that "often used forms of treatment, such as pain medications, physical therapy, and chiropractic treatment, are not effective for a large portion of the fibromyalgia populations" (pp. 41-48). Long further states that Noller and Sprott (2003) showed that these therapies produced no improvement in pain over a two-year period. Also, that (Baumgartner et al. 2002) showed that in follow-up of fibromyalgia patients six years after the initial evaluation the symptoms of fibromyalgia persisted.

According to Rooks (2007) recent studies support the recommendation of a multimodal approach to treatment involving individualized, evidence-based pharmacotherapy and self-management. Treatment goals should include the improvement of symptoms, primarily pain and sleep, and the promotion of positive health behaviors with the aim of improving physical function and emotional wellbeing. "Additionally, the development of a core group of outcome measures would allow appropriate comparison of interventions and the fast development of a uniform standard of care for this population" (pp. 111-117).

Molton, Graham, Stoelb, and Jensen (2007) prove a review of the rationale and evidence supporting three frequently used psychosocial interventions for chronic pain: cognitive-behavioral therapy, operant behavioral therapy, and self-hypnosis training.

Recent clinical trials and laboratory work continue to support the use of cognitive behavioral therapy and operant behavioral therapy as adjunctive treatments for chronic pain. Self-hypnosis training can provide temporary pain relief to the majority of individuals with chronic pain. Cognitive-behavioral therapy and operant behavioral therapy treatments focus on factors that exacerbate or maintain suffering in chronic pain, and should be considered as part of a multidisciplinary treatment paradigm be explored to aid in the self-healing process.

"Smile and laugh every chance you get. Smiles and laughter infuse your body with healing chemistry and lighten your mood and that of others."
― *Marcia Emery*

Chapter 5. What is the Pain Experience?

As I have explained previously, the body's internal chemicals, the neuropeptides and their receptors, are the actual biological underpinnings of awareness, manifesting themselves as emotions, beliefs, and expectations, and profoundly influencing how one responds to and experiences their world.

Over the years, I have listened as female clients, who are dealing with chronic conditions, especially fibromyalgia, tell a similar story. They feel alone and misunderstood. They are fighting a battle every day to deal with pain, and yet they try to appear somewhat normal to those around them. They complain that most of their family and friends think they are dramatizing their condition, or even trying to neglect themselves or responsibilities, because others do not understand the intensity of their afflictions.

Many researchers have explored chronic pain condition causes and medical, nutritional, and complementary medicine approaches to alleviate symptoms, but little has been explored regarding the self-talk used to improve the condition. Nor, have they explored the effectiveness of this information being used with patients with severe symptoms, especially if they are also in a state of despair or depression. Quantitative data regarding fibromyalgia shows that different methods and treatments produce different results in patients with few successful approaches. However, knowledge of all of the possibilities enables a fibromyalgia patient to try various options or combinations of options to improve their condition. Quality of life data are also very important to provide the patient with comprehensive information about positive potential health. This will also provide information for the healthcare community to assist fibromyalgia patients from all backgrounds, in making improvements.

The thoughts and questions that led to the development of this study were:

- An individual is living with the experience of the disease of Fibromyalgia (FM) and despairs of feeling better and having a healthier lifestyle. While not immediately life threatening, the diagnosis carries the weight of major lifestyle changes with the possibility of curtailing many activities.
- The individual may have a "defeatist" attitude, and the mindset of succumbing to life as a semi-invalid. There may be feelings of helplessness or depression, and an acceptance of the prognosis. He or she may lack the desire to seek out other opinions, or alternative health care options. Health care providers may offer little hope of recovering or even alleviating their symptoms.
- Yet many individuals do start to think about trying something to improve their situation. What self-talk took place to make this change in their thinking? This research study explores what the change in that communication is, and how that change came to take place. The specific research aim of the study was: What is the experience of

women living with fibromyalgia who have been improving their health? What methods, both mental and physical, were employed to realize a level of healing? What research has been conducted in the area of mind-body healing?

A qualitative phenomenological approach was employed to analyze the experiences of the women participating in the study. Creswell (1998) explains that phenomenological researchers depend almost exclusively on lengthy interviews with a carefully selected sample of participants, all of whom have had direct experience with the phenomenon being studied. Harmon (1991) emphasized that "whereas we learn certain kinds of things from distancing ourselves from the subject studied, we get another kind of knowledge from intuitively 'becoming one with' the subject. We do not learn about reality from controlled experiments but rather by identifying with the observed" (pp. 50-55).

Byrne (2001) explains that phenomenological researchers hope to gain understanding of the essential "truths" of the lived experience. The term phenomenology often is used without a clear understanding of its meaning. "Phenomenology has been described as a philosophy, methodology, and method. Knowledge and understanding are embedded in our everyday world, but cannot be quantified or reduced to numbers of statistics. Phenomenologists believe that truth and understanding of life can emerge from people's lived experiences" (p. 830).

According to Moustakas (1994) in phenomenological studies the researcher abstains from making supposition, focuses on a specific topic freshly and naively, constructs a question or problem to guide the study, and derives findings that will provide the basis for further research and reflection.

The individual then constructs a full description of his or her conscious experience. This is the textural description and includes thoughts, feelings, examples, ideas, and situations that portray what comprises an experience. The challenge is to explicate the phenomenon in terms of its constituents and possible meanings, thus discerning the features of consciousness and arriving at an understanding of the essences of the experience.

I was interested in what internal dialogue occurred in a fibromyalgia patient that encouraged her to seek changes in her health, and were these same dialogues common among all or most of the women who had realized better change of health? Therefore, this method would provide an understanding of the quality of their lives, and commonalties of the self-talk among them.

In the process of these interviews, I expected that various themes would emerge, and again, would the same circumstances or various individual circumstances cause each woman to arrive at the same health decisions. Moreover, were these decisions the same or extremely individualized?

Each participant was asked the same four open-ended questions. The replies varied from terse, factual answers to rich, descriptive and often emotional narratives. While most of the narratives included feelings of frustration and helplessness in the body's ability to deal with the disease, the reasons for making a change and the methods used to realize those changes were varied and innovative. I noted the perseverance and creativity that were common characteristics among these women.

The study was conducted using oral, qualitative, unstructured interviews with each participant. Audio tapes were used to record their narratives while they described their experience with fibromyalgia. I asked four open-ended questions about: (1) their history with fibromyalgia, (2) the experience of being diagnosed, (3) making a change, and (4) living the experience. I was looking for what self-talk may have occurred to change their attitude and belief system regarding the disease, and their determination to make some change in their health. I was also looking for their present condition and their present mindset. I extracted and systematically organized their narratives, concentrating on the reflections and descriptions of the experiences provided by each individual.

Documenting the common themes that emerged and clearly identifying them provided a detailed and integrated description of the human experience of living with fibromyalgia, as well as eliciting the self-talk and lifestyle changes that led each individual to realize improved health.

The study further shows the necessity of intrapersonal communication for neuro-connective healing. It asks the question: What types of self-communication were most effective to motivate women with fibromyalgia to make a positive change to affect their health?

In recruiting participants the recruitment criteria was as follows:
- Diagnosed with fibromyalgia.
- 1 year of feeling some degree of (self-assessed) improved health.
- Age: 35 – 65
- Gender: women
- Willing to meet with the researcher and give an interview.

I had a very difficult time recruiting participants. A recruitment notice was posted on the website and in the newsletter of the Greater Chicago Chapter of the Arthritis Foundation, the Fibromyalgia website, my church bulletin, and I asked many friends and acquaintances for referrals. In addition, whenever

I represented the Arthritis Foundation at Health Fairs or gave presentations and talks during this time, I was always recruiting. Not only did most of the women who admitted to having fibromyalgia say no; many of them actually took a physical step backwards. And the answers were usually a version of "I do not think I can do that." I always explained the small amount of time involved, the promise of anonymity and the importance to me to conduct this study.

And yet, of the perhaps close to 100 women that were asked, only 15 could be recruited. One of these possible participants backed out, and another I had to drop because she did not provide enough of an answer to the questions, and therefore, did not give me any data with which to work. Fifteen participants or respondents met the inclusion criteria and fourteen of them gave IRB approved informed consent. One of these was eliminated because of lack of depth.

Methods

After recruiting the interviewees, appointments were made. Most of the interviews were conducted in the individual's homes. All of the interviews were conducted one-on-one, using four open-ended questions, and audio taped. I did little if any talking except perhaps to repeat a question or ask for further clarification. Each tape was assigned a coded number, which became that participant's study number for files also. Each narrative was then analyzed for important or recurring word phrases and themes. All of the narratives were then analyzed for the recurrent and common underlying themes among them to form a pattern.

Patterns

As part of the analytical process I developed individual themes and then patterns. The themes were topics of conversation or word phrases the participants used in narrating their experiences with fibromyalgia. These were either recurring phrases, or places in the narrative upon which the participant placed particular emphasis, or passion in relating her experience.

I then listed every expression relevant to the experience, and included recurring words or phrases. Expressions not meeting these requirements were eliminated. Preliminary grouping was performed to cluster and thematize by giving each of these a numeric category relating to:

1. Lifestyle
2. History
3. Methods tried
4. Coping skills
5. Present thinking/condition

In the next step of the analytical process, I then developed patterns consisting of the recurrence of themes among all of the participants. It consisted of similar content or similar phraseology among the individual themes. I listed all of the participant's analyses and began to form a depiction of the commonalties of all of the participants. I then summarized the most common phrases and themes divested from each participant's individually analyzed narrative.

The following list begins to show emerging patterns and themes.

Commonalities Among Participants

Number of Ladies	Commonalties in their Narratives
13	Have other physical/medical conditions
13	Feel people/doctors do not understand
12	Physical problems /medicines and Concern about dependency
11	Rest, conserve energy, prioritize activities, set limits
11	Use inner strength, positive people, Positive attitude, spiritual
11	Creative in methods: exercise, stretch, acupuncture, meditation, magnets, heat
11	Use phrases like: mind over matter, just get on with it, work through it /ignore pain
10	Refuse to give in/right attitude
10	Lived with pain, stress most of life
10	Believe knowledge of disease important
7	Need/believe can control condition
4	Physically abused or raped
4	Fatalistic, not much one can do

Analysis of All Participants

Participants, Age, Profile/Lifestyle, Approximate Years with Fibromyalgia, Other Chronic Conditions.

6-0330 No-show for interview

Aster. 35 Caucasian,
Married,
Office worker
10-15 years
Fibromyalgia, arthritis, depression

This participant indicated at the time I was arranging an interview that she was better than in the past. She was very reluctant to give information and believed that nothing she had to say would be worth contributing. She gets no support from family or friends and has tried several options to no avail. She is resigned to the state of her condition. She had to be dropped from the study.

Blossom. 64 Afro-American Single
1 grown male child
10 years
Diabetes

She had to cut back on activities and group volunteering because of the pain. She was diagnosed by several psychologists and put on strong meds that caused many dangerous incidents, one almost fatal. She has analyzed her condition, and limitations, and manages her days in the way that works for that particular day. She believes "you gotta do what you gotta do."

Dahlia. 65 Caucasian
Married, second
Grown children
Over 10 years ago
Rheumatoid & Osteo Arthritis

Attributes a lot of her health problems to being married to an abusive husband, who actually tried to kill her. She has many problems/other physical conditions along with fibromyalgia. She has a lot of pain, is sensitive to many medications, and does not feel pain is being managed as well as it could be. She is very concerned about her limitations, and wants to be as active as she once was. She is rather fatalistic; believing there is not much more she can do. However, she does read and search the internet for more information. She also believes in ignoring the pain as much as possible and just hanging in there and going along with it.

Daisy. 65 Caucasian
Divorced
Medical professional – cytologist.
Runs a small boarding house.
Unknown, Came on in middle-age
Diabetic, high blood pressure, hypothyroidism, stroke,
Fredrickson IV, Lipohyperdia,
Bi-polar disorder, arterial-sclerosis

She had a healthy childhood and middle age. She refers numerous times to her age and attributes a lot of her FM and other medical conditions, to her age. She tried many medications and has problems mixing them with her various medical conditions. She paces her activities, hires help when she needs it and meditates a lot. She has found ways to accept and deal with her condition and remain relatively comfortable. However, she also seemed to have a defeatist or fatalistic attitude. But this seems to serve her well and contributes to her comfort.

Flora. 63 Caucasian
Single
Retired office worker,
Volunteer with several organizations
Had pain & problems since age 20.
Diagnosed at age 50
Hypothyroidism, Hasimoto thyroidism, osteoarthritis

She has lived with pain all of her life, some of it very severe. She questions the physical abuse her mother endured during pregnancy with her as contributing to her condition. She has been very creative and diligent in finding ways to treat herself. She believes she has to keep control of her condition, and with God's help she can.

Heather. 56 Caucasian
Single
Mental Health Therapist
About 8-9 years
Diagnosed 5 years ago.
Osteoarthritis, golfers elbow, tendonitis of right thumb

Has had a lot of trauma in her life. She was raped at an early age, has lost all; of her relatives, and some friends to death. She has several physical conditions she is dealing with. She relied primarily on medications to manage her various conditions. Tried magnets, laughter, and denial of pain and physical restrictions to cope with these conditions. She believes her faith in god and her attitude are important parts of her living successfully with FM. She admits to being somewhat fatalistic, and that she

has grown and changed because of her experience
       She has empathy and compassion for those less fortunate than her, and counts her blessings.

> **Hyacinth. 54** Caucasian
>   Married, daughter in college, teacher
>   Approximately 10 years
>   Scoliosis

       She feels support and love from her medical team and her family and friends. She had a broken ankle, surgery, was a caregiver, and had miscellaneous pains for many years. Best treatment was medication for sleep and acupuncture. Then she could exercise and does that regularly. Knew she had to help herself, had to make lifestyle changes. Believes in being persistent, doing research, having faith, and discovering what specifically works for them you.

> **Iris. 55** Caucasian
>   Divorced
>   Grown children
>   Past nurse, Office worker
>   Had symptoms 15-18 years
>   Diagnosed possibly 5 years ago
>   Chronic Fatigue, Migraines, Thyroid problems

       As a former nurse she has strong health analyzing abilities. She has had a lot of stress, caregiving, and anger issues for most of her life. She feels those issues have contributed to her ill health. She did a lot of research, reading, and moving around from practitioner to practitioner to find answers and relief. She has adjusted her attitude and continues to adjust it. She is very critical about herself.

Ivy. 63 Caucasian
Divorced
Grown children
Nurse
7-8 years
COPD, tendonitis, hypothyroid, Sjogren syndrome, inflammatory rheumatism

She was in and out of pain since a child. Was told by her mother at an early age that she was a chronic complainer. She learned to live with pain and "Just get on with it." She is used to doing what must be done regardless of pain. She copes by living within limitations. Believes treatments for her hypothyroid condition is helping her FM condition. Would really like to be touched and hugged without pain.

Jasmine. 58 Caucasian
Married
3 grown boys
Psychotherapist
15 years
Myofascial syndrome,
Osteoarthritis,
possible paget's disease,
hyperparathyroid

She learned to ignore pain and not rest until she had no choice because she could not keep going. She has many complicated conditions and numerous surgeries. She has had many problems with medications. She defines herself as an optimist. And she knows that she can ignore things and go ahead and accomplish what she has to do, but only for a period of time. She has learned over the years to rest, use heat, and stretches. She is spiritual and uses imagery, self-hypnosis, affirmations, and belief in God as part of her coping skills. She continues to seek medical and alternative methods and answers to deal with her various conditions.

Lily. 41 Caucasian
Married,
2 small boys
Part-time Hair dresser,
and Greeting card company
11 years
TMJ

Is determined not to be a victim of FM. She researches information, therapies, medications, and self-help routines to find relief. She is realistic about her limitations, and believes that attitude and acceptance are an important part of living successfully with FM. She also believes that communication with doctors and other relationships in her life is important.

Petunia. 37 Caucasian
Married
Psychotherapist
10 years
Arthritis, TMJ, migraines, sinus

She was diagnosed at an early age. She feels she must have control over her condition and lifestyle. She is concerned about depending on medication and prefers to use exercise and holistic methods to manage her condition. She tries to stay around positive people and keep positive thoughts. She also believes knowledge and the right attitude imbues the power to control symptoms. She sees herself as a strong person with a strong will and refuses to give in to the disease. She has become more aware of her needs, and got tired of complaining. And she told herself that you have to do your part if you want to get better, but she sometimes feels like she is handicapped.

Rose. 41 Caucasian
Married, 1 boy
Poly-soma
12 years
Arthritis, asthma, GERD, hypothyroidism, hypertension

Once she was on the meds and started feeling a little better, she got out of her initial rut. When she found a doctor who believed in her and knew what he was doing she had an ally she could go to, and began believing there were things that she could do or things that would help her. She realized she could not continue living the way that she was living, needed to get some help, and then needed to change her attitude in order to cope and live with the fibromyalgia.

Violet. 65 Caucasian
Married, grown children
2nd marriage
Past office worker
Had problems in early twenties.
Diagnosed approx 13 years ago.
Arthritis, Chronic Fatigue

She has learned to conserve her energy and therefore is able to do more than before. She prioritizes her activities, whether tasks or fun, and forces herself to do them. She refuses to give up/give in, uses her inner strength, and is doing better. She used phrases like: make myself, push myself, mind over matter and I cope because that's my mindset.

"No matter what happens with this illness, I think it is possible to carve out a dignified and productive life from it".
- Laura Hillenbrand

Chapter 6. Discussion and Interpretation
Discussion:

From this analysis, the I recognized that though all of the participant's personalities and experiences were unique, six core themes emerged that characterized the experience of living with fibromyalgia and getting better for the participants in this study. These themes are:

♦ **Comorbid Conditions.** All of the participants had other physical or medical conditions, and most had problems with medicines and were concerned about dependency on medications.

♦ **Lack of Trust**. Disbelief and/or lack of trust as the participants feel that people, especially the medical field, but also friends and family members, who do not understand fibromyalgia and their experience of living with it.

♦ **Self-care**. Participants learned to manage their physical problems and their personal lives by conserving energy and prioritizing activities.

♦ **Inner Strength**. Some women described this as spiritual strength.

♦ **Alternative Therapies**. Participants reported using complementary and alternative therapies: such as acupuncture, meditation, and magnets, to name a few.

♦ **Perseverance**. Self-talk was used as a means of self-support as they persisted in their search for relief from their symptoms.

Comorbid Conditions.
All of the participants had other medical physical conditions; the most prevalent were different types of thyroid problems. The next prevalent was arthritis, and then there were a range of conditions including diabetes, migraines, TMJ and 8 3 chronic fatigue. They had concerns regarding the medications that were prescribed for the fibromyalgia and these coexisting conditions.

Examples are:

- "I take aspirin that helps. I've been given all the N-saids that were ever invented. And I have had also the worst side effects… If you name it, I've been on it, and they make me sicker, and do not take away any of my muscle pain, nor my foot pain. None of the medications the doctors put me on work. Prednisone worked the best, but I worry about the side effects on the liver and kidneys."
- "I tried all these antidepressants which are supposedly a painkiller. None of those worked. I was later put on naproxin, nothing."
- "I went to a doctor because of pain in my hip thinking maybe it was the bone and he said let's try prednisone. Well, my heart was pounding, I thought I was having a heart attack

one time. Right now I'm on a muscle relaxant. It's not helping. When I take a half pill of remaran and a half pill of klonapin I tend to sleep."

- "I went through a lot of medications that helped some, but not a lot. After a while I started feeling like a guinea pig and I was gaining a little weight. I think I'm too young to be relying on medicine. And I don't think they really know what it does to you in the long term. I worry about that. I worry about my liver and kidneys and cancer, and this build-up of junk in my system."

Lack of Trust.

All of the participants expressed concern that their doctors and friends and family did not understand what they were experiencing.

Examples are:

- "I brought an article to the doctor and I said: 'gee, could I have this, 'cause I have all the symptoms?' He said: 'well yes, but you're not the personality for it'."

- "They're running tests, and running tests, and scratching their heads, and they're telling me that I'm depressed. And (finally) it became recognized as a disease, but the doctors didn't recognize it. They just said: 'oh, that's just something that they put a name to, to give you all something to say, but it's really all just in your head. You're depressed and you're having some mental problems. See a psychologist'."

- "So I went to doctors and some of them I think really didn't get that all the symptoms were together. And when I found somebody that did, I was kind of relieved that they put a name to it. They actually said, yeah, it's not all in your head. Even though they still at the time kind of alluded to – well if you take antidepressants, you'll just be better. And, you know, it's kind of like a neurotic physical condition, that women have or something."

- "It would just be so nice if everyone would understand, because you don't have something on the outside. Because no one knows, you can't feel that my arms, everything from my head to my toes hurts."
- "I heard a lot of: you don't look handicapped. You're not, and yet there are days when I feel like it."
- "Once you have it and have it for long enough, people get sick of your complaining and hearing about how you feel, so you don't talk about it, you just deal with it."

Self-care.

The women in this study were creative and determined to find ways to manage their condition and improve their quality of life.

Examples are:

- "I think you probably learn what your limitations are. Learn that, because once you can learn that, then you can take care of yourself better. When you need to rest, you rest. If you need to cancel something, you cancel. Because you don't feel good. You don't just keep pushing, pushing all the time. And that's what most people do. They don't want to accept that they have a limitation maybe and so if they push themselves hard enough they think they can overcome kind of on their own, and they can't."
- "I try to sleep better, I do try to eat better, I just kinda do what I've gotta do. One way of taking care of myself was switching jobs. If I were free of the health problem, I would clean the

house from top to bottom. Which I am trying in bits and pieces but I just wear out."

- "I know that I'm limited, that's why I don't wear myself out with insignificant things. You know, like cleaning the house every day or doing something like that. So I limit myself. And I save my energy for what I'm going to do. I'll try to lay around a little bit more when I know I'm going out that evening."

Inner/Spiritual Strength.

The commonality of inner strength or spirituality the participants expressed as one of the inner resources ways that they developed of taking care of themselves.

Examples are:

- "I've always had prayer in my life, but I have even more so. And people will say, how can you live like this here? Aren't you angry? And I say no, because God has shown me the way to take care of myself."
- "Spiritually, I have strong faith, and I believe that God walks with me in everything. And I can do all things through He who strengthens me. So, I continue to do. It's an action verb."
- "I feel very close to God, and I was raised in the Unity church …I was raised with affirmations. I was raised with affirming my health. I was raised with affirming my relationship with God and all creation "
- "There was one time I came home, in March or whenever it was when we had that freaky snow, and the trees hadn't had all their leaves on or anything, and just all the snow on it. It was just gorgeous. So when I drive through there it's just like: 'Thank you, God, that was so nice.'

Yeah, things like that kind of keep me going. Things that just make me smile inside."

Alternative Therapies.

These women all realized they would have to find their own answers. Whether it was seeking other medical professionals, trying alternative methods, and/or changing treatment practices that were no longer effective for them.

Examples are:

- "My inner healing resource is to gain knowledge about my disease processes. And learning about them, I have learned to deal with a lot of this without my doctor's help. I don't wear high heels or tight clothing."
- "I would go for a manipulations, probably once a week. I got a dog; I got a four-legged furry therapist. I've had massage therapy, and I have my regimen of heat, stretching and rest. I use heat packs. I do imagery. If it's real hard for me to focus and the pain level is high, it seems like when I start praying for other people that I can focus on that and then I start relaxing. I also have this technique that I focus on parts of my body that don't hurt. And I think it comes from doing self-hypnosis. I'm trained in clinical hypnosis."
- "I tried nutrition therapy, acupuncture, colonics, electronic footbaths, and injections of high dosage of vitamins and minerals, and fluids (similar to hyperallementation). Bufferin, massage therapy, and sauna are the three things that help or make me feel comfortable."
- "I went to a napropath, tried Rolfing, and started exercising. But acupuncture and Chinese herbs helped me the most."
- "I found isometrics work best. I use heat patches and massage my scalp

with a plastic brush to control my pain. I have used paraffin wax treatment for the stiffness and trigger finger."

Perseverance.
Self-talk helped them to persevere. Examples are:
- "I have learned to ignore it, believe it or not. And if things hurt, I just kinda cuss under my breath and just keep moving."
- "One of the things I have been trying to tell myself is that I am happy, I am healthy, I am well. Every day in every way I'm getting better and better. And my cells are happy and my cells are well."
- "I said things like: this can't continue, I can't live like this, I refuse to live like this forever. Because if this is how I have to live the quality of life is bad, I don't like it. And I just refused to totally give in to it. Because I know I have more control over things. I can't get rid of it; there's no cure for it. Even if I can't make myself physically feel better by exercising or whatever. I can still approach it mentally from the perspective that I can still control how I want to respond to it."
- "I think you just accept the fact that you have it and it's something that you're going to deal with the rest of your life. You are still going to have it; you're still going to have problems. But once you get past that I think it's just easier to deal with. As long as I can maintain my own then I won't let other people take advantage of me so much. So that has helped a lot. I say it different in my head but 'kiss my butt' attitude is what I would call it. So it's almost like you stand up for yourself a little bit more. And that's better for me, instead of being the doormat."

- "You're going to be in pain, ok. If I'm going to hurt, whether I'm doing something or not, then I might as well do something and have fun. So, I didn't let it stop me. I just have goals in life and one of my goals in life is to make somebody laugh every day. Laughter is healing mechanism. I feel if I'm sick or something, I haven't been laughing enough."

"There is only one true path to your wellness, that is the one that you choose and you shape as you travel upon it."
- G. Sprissler

Interpretation of the Study

Many of the women in the study went to several doctors before they were accurately diagnosed. And many were told that there was little or nothing that could be done about their condition. Sobel (2000) reports the story of a woman who goes to see a third doctor after many months of suffering from numbness and weakness that was severe one day and nonexistent the next. The symptoms were not confined to one area, traveling to different body parts. The first two doctors had told her, "It's all in your head," at worst making the condition sound like a figment of her imagination and at best suggesting that she was not effectively managing the stresses of everyday life. The new doctor did a complete workup and extensive testing at the end of which she was told she had multiple sclerosis, an incurable disease that can slowly destroy the nervous system, eventually causing death.

But when the doctor told her this diagnosis, she responded, "Oh, I'm so relieved, I thought it was all in my head." I heard this same type of relief filled story over and over again from the participants. "I was so glad to finally get a diagnosis, even though I didn't like it." "I was told or I thought it was all in my head."

Caudill, Schnable, Zuttermeister, Benson and Friedman (1991) and other researchers collaborated on a study of the effects of mind/body/ medicine on patients with chronic pain trying to gain relief from pain. Caudill introduced HMO patients to the relaxation response, exercise, nutrition, and stress management in weekly meetings that lasted for ten weeks. She found that after one year there was a 36% reduction in clinic visits among these patients – an estimated net savings of $12,000 (Caudill et al. 1991).

In a similar study Hellman, Budd, Borysenko, McClelland, and Hendricks (2007) achieved a 50% reduction in office visits at another HMO with primary care patients. Another important component in healing is mindfulness. When the mind is in a context, the body is necessarily also in that context. To achieve a different physiological state, sometimes what we need to do is to place the mind in another context. Thus, the different state of mind means a different state for the body (Langer, 1990).

Mindfulness focuses on inquiring into our experience of the present moment, and being receptive to what arises. It is the nonjudgmental attention to experiences in the present moment. It typically cultivates in a formal practice such as sitting meditation, walking meditation, or mindful movements. It is bringing consciousness into whatever we are doing such as looking at something, or smelling something or touching something and really experiencing what it looks, or smells or feels like. It is the single-minded awareness of what is happening to us and in us at successive moments of perception.

In intentionally connecting with our unfolding experience the attitude that is being cultivated is one of being open to, accepting and being present to whatever arises for us in the moment, without having to fix it or try to get rid of it (Kabat-Zinn, 2005). The main ways that mindfulness improves our quality of life is attention regulation, body awareness, emotion regulation and sense of self. These factors synergistically create a sense of calm and wellbeing.

Santorelli (1992) suggests that mindfulness can be described as the cultivation of one's inherent capacity to fluidity and flexibility by paying attention to physical and mental status non-judgmentally from moment to moment. Meditation can be defined as paying attention on purpose for self-understanding. Mindfulness meditation is a highly refined, systematic attentional strategy to develop both calmness of mind and body and deep insight into varied mental and physical conditions that inhibit our capacity to respond proactively and effectively in demanding more commonplace everyday activities.

Meili and Kabat-Zinn (2004) explain that all of us regularly need to learn to live inside ourselves again to one degree or another because things are constantly changing. As we age, our bodies and our minds are going through all sorts of changes.

Learning to live inside again and to deal with how things are becomes something of a lifetime adventure, but you have to be open to it. You have to be sensitive to working up to your limits and then listening very, very carefully. Letting the give and the take happen to you through your body and your mind until you feel the next level emerge. We are beginning to uncover evidence suggesting that the mind can influence healing in human beings. And while this science is in its infancy, the potential clinical value of the fact itself is huge. Medicine will be more participatory medicine in the 21st century.

When we consider the full capacity of one's own inward being, the capacity to learn to listen, learn, grow and sense, and thereby feel, heal, and then grow again; that is something that is a lifetime work to refine and develop and grow into.

A study conducted by Morone, Lynch, Greco,

Tindle and Weiner (2008) on older adults with chronic low back pain showed several themes reflecting the beneficial effects of mindfulness meditation. Several themes were identified related to pain reduction, improved attention, improved sleep, and achieving well-being resulting from mindfulness meditation that suggest it has promising potential as a nonpharmacologic treatment of chronic pain for older adults.

Battino (2000) discusses the "Swish" Technique, which is named for a change occurring as fast as you say "Whsst", and is based on guided visualization using submodalities. Submodalities are ways that our brains sort and code our experience. Within the visual modality, like making a picture in your mind, the submodalities would include: color, distance, size, depth, clarity, contrast, scope, intensity of hue, moving or static, speed of movement, aspect ratio or proportion, orientation, whether bounded or famed, tilt, and foreground, background relationship. These are ways in which you can alter an image. Visual imagery is preferred since it is relatively easy within the mind to work with two or three visual submodalities at the same time – it is difficult to do this for kinesthetic and auditory.

The Swish Technique is a kind of behavior modification approach where the brain is programmed to replace one image or depiction of yourself with another. The repetition and speed are important so that you achieve an almost automatic replacement of how you perceive yourself. Brains can learn very rapidly.

McCracken, Gauntlett-Gilbert and Vowles (2007) define mindfulness as a quality of behavior that includes full, non-reactive, accepting, and present-focused awareness of experience. They explain that clinical methods of mindfulness and the processes that underlie them appear to have clear implications for chronic pain, but have not been rigorously investigated to this point in time. The purpose of this study was to examine mindfulness in relation to the pain, emotional, physical, and social functioning of individuals with chronic pain. In each instance greater mindfulness was associated with better functioning. When disease is thought to be purely physiological and incurable it may be more amenable to individual control than humans have believed in the past. Even when the disease progresses unrelentingly, one's reactions to it can be mindful or mindless and change its impact on them.

    Langer (1990) points this out in her book on mindfulness. Langer goes on to explain that paying attention to vague feelings, is a way to have a dialogue with this inner body sense and accessing the body's experiences of meaning. It provides the opportunity to gain new insights, and physical release or bodily shift. She also describes two ways in which humans have learned to influence health: exchanging unhealthy mindsets for healthy ones and increasing a generally mindful state. The latter is more lasting and results in more personal control. Humans control their health, or the course of their disease, without really knowing that they do. Now they may be able to learn how to recognize and use their control over illness. They need to consider things from multiple perspectives.

    Mindfulness leads to feelings of control, greater freedom of action, and less burnout. I discovered that the most common characteristic among the women in this study was that they had one or more other conditions along with the fibromyalgia. Almost all had problems with some or all of the medications that were prescribed for them. All of the participants were very creative in finding a way to live with fibromyalgia, and/or to alleviate the symptoms of this condition. Many expressed a refusal to give-in and the importance of adapting the right attitude to deal with it. And for many they have either lived with a lot of pain or stressful conditions for most of their life. Eleven out of the 13 women learned to take rest periods and conserve their energy. And, 11 of them said they used inner strength, positive thoughts, and are spiritual.

All healing is first spiritual healing, from radiation therapy to antidepressant medication, according to Mehl-Madrona (2003). He serves as Medical Director at the Center for Complementary Medicine and Faculty/Residency Programs at the University of Pittsburgh Medical Center. Healing the spirit is necessary to heal the body. Treatment fails when one does not do this. The soul must give permission for physical manipulation, surgery, and drugs to succeed. This helps to further one's therapies. Resistance weakens one's efforts, makes their antibiotics ineffective, and prevents surgical incisions from healing.

Mehl-Madrona (2003) also states that conflict is inherent to most adventures. If healing is an adventure, obstacles and adversaries are to be expected. "Illness presents itself as an obstacle to our plans. …Healing is a struggle. We must externalize the enemy – the illness. We must cast it out of ourselves and create a dialogue in which we gain the upper hand and force it to transform into healthy cells. Or to depart from our midst" (p. 19).

Over half of all Americans believe that their religious faith helped them recover from injury, illness or disease (McNichol, 1996). Patients know how important spirituality is in their treatment, so do many physicians. Although spirituality is routinely ignored as a relevant part of a medical history or a psychological assessment (Miller, 1997). Spirituality refers to the relationship and belief system a person has with the transcendent aspects of being. Thus spirituality may underlay, but is not synonymous with, religion. It also may or may not include a formal "belief in God." It does include a belief or felt experience of an aspect of life that is more than material, emotional or mental. This may be felt as experience of a greater creative principle in nature, belief in intrinsic purpose and meaning, or an expanded sense of the self (Targ, 2000).

Several of the participants stated that they felt spiritual in some way, but were not necessarily religious.

The next theme that emerged was that the women prioritized activities, set limits, and believed that seeking out information is crucial. They also needed to feel that they could control their condition. And this encouraged them to continue to adjust their lifestyles in order to cope and be active.

Pelletier (1994) emphasizes that control is the conviction that individuals can affect the course and destiny of their lives. Once an individual voluntarily or involuntarily experiences a deep sense of inner strength or personal control, even in the midst of major trauma, that experience becomes the core of a mature sense of personal empowerment and control.

Recent research shows that this factor of control, empowerment, or self-efficacy may be the ultimate determinant in human health and even aging. Sullivan (1991) U.S. Secretary of Health and Human Services explains: Personal responsibility, which is to say responsible and enlightened behavior by each and every individual, truly is the key to good health. Man has become increasingly health-conscious; increasingly appreciative of the extent to which their physical and emotional well-being is dependent upon that only they, themselves, can affect" (pp. 291-297).

Nunley (1999) suggests that true healing seldom involves putting things back like they were before dysfunction or disease. Healing requires moving forward. Consequently, healing is always a transformational, integrative process that carries one forward. And there must be room for spontaneity, creativity, and improvisation. I agree that healing is assuredly an integrative process, therefore the subtheme of this undertaking. I also suggest that any time anyone is faced with decisions to change their lifestyle or change what they are doing about things, there are really two parts of the process, which are the "how" and the "why" of it. The "how" is the mechanics, the "why" is the dynamics of it. And, when one talks of lifestyle changes, one is not just talking about setting limitations, eating, and exercising but that there has to be a values change, and a priority change within to make it permanent. One has to examine what they are doing and how it affects them to see where their priorities are, and to set out a game plan of where they want to go with it.

    I believe the concern of the participants in this study was not so much the quantity of their remaining life, but with the quality and the loss of the potential abilities in that life. I think that small goals were set and that the participants asked themselves: If I do this, will it help a little? What if I try a few other things? What combination of things seems to be working? And from time to time, what modifications and adjustments have to be made?

    Why did these women decide to try something to get better? Some said that "this is the worst I've ever been, I don't want to get any worse." They were at the bottom. Others believed that: "if being where I am hurts, it can't hurt much worse to try, and even if it causes more pain I'm still going to try." Many knew that they have been unwell several times and got better, so they wanted to try to repeat the process. They have proven in the past that it was possible, so they believed it was possible to do it again. Was the belief system or the releasing of a holding pattern or both the foundation for healing?

    According to Taylor (1997) one of the most important contributions that mind/body medicine has to make in the vast array of alternative and complementary healing systems now in practice is the role of consciousness in healing. What does one need to know to harness the patient's beliefs for healing? It means looking for a phenomenological, existential, intuitive, and dynamic psychology of inner experience that the individual has constructed to understand reality, rather than treating the patient's beliefs as mere cognitive thought processes to be measured.

Individuals who have experienced an opening of the internal doors of perception and committed themselves to a life-long journey of interior exploration have generally already constructed a sophisticated psychological language of inner experience as a way to navigate the interior domains of consciousness they have experienced.

Warter points out that we find ourselves at a critical time of convergence and integration of healing modalities which bring back into relevance and focus the importance of our spirituality for the living and healing process. A greater number of healthcare practitioners and healers are incorporating this into their practices and approaches to healing. It has been demonstrated that the religious and spiritual belief systems, inner experiences, and world vision of both the patient and the physician are clinically relevant and provide assistance in preventing physical and mental illness.

These factors are also significant for the patient in understanding, coping and recovering from illness. More and more interest in the spiritual aspects of healing is emerging within traditional healthcare disciplines and there are many new innovative training programs that address the spiritual perspective of the lives of patients and healers in the healing process (Warter, 2000).

The purpose of a study conducted by Sharoff (2008) was to describe the experience that holistic nurses have in incorporating complementary and alternative modalities in the care of their clients. Also, to gain a deeper understanding of holistic nurses and the perceived benefit of utilizing a holistic modality with their clients and themselves concurrently as providers of these modalities. She had six conclusions. First, holistic nurses have awareness of what they need to foster their own growth and development. Second, they are open and willing to explore different modalities of the healing-caring process for themselves. Third, they are committed to maintaining congruency between personal needs and professional goals and ethics. Fourth, is the concept of caring for one's self. Fifth is that the nurse-client relationship is fundamental the healing-caring process of both the nurse and the client. Finally, benefits to client's continued health promotion and comfort care are integral to the healing-caring process. The findings of this study can be used to further the understanding and appreciation of both holistic nursing and the holistic nurse.

According to Wisneski (1997) there is a need for western allopathic medicine to expand its current concepts of anatomy to include the human energy field, which is the foundation of Chinese and Indian medicine systems and of certain intuitive healers. This human energy field interacts with other ambient fields, including the fields of all other living organisms.

Crucial to understanding the physiology of the human energy field is the role of the endocrine glands, in particular the pineal gland, which act as energy transducers. These glands/energy transducers convert external energy, which impinges upon the human field in a variety of forms (light, sound, etc.) into electrical and then chemical energy in the form of hormones and peptides. He also suggests that expression of relaxation hormones (melatonin, endorphins, etc.) may occur when the brain is vibrating in alpha wave frequencies. The unified energy field theory of physiology becomes a bridge to a new medical paradigm, an integrated medicine that unites eastern and western concepts of the human body, and other systems of healing and wellness medicine.

As explained earlier in this book by Ader (1981) Lipton (2005) and Pert (1997), negative thoughts and emotions release harmful chemicals through the system weakening cell structure and the immune system. Positive thoughts and emotions release healthful and healing chemicals strengthening cellular structure and the immune system.

In a stressed situation the body is protected from mortal assault, but at the same time is left remarkably vulnerable, according to Wisneski (1997). A study of medical students (Glaser & Kiecolt-Glaser, 2005) showed that on the first day of final exams, their levels of circulating lymphocytes were diminished. Under stress, the lymphocytes receive a hormonal turn-off signal. A survival mechanism has misinterpreted the life-threatening nature of the stressor. For now, it remains to be seen just how far-reaching the effect of a stressful life can be on an individual's wellness.

Wisneski (1999) adds that "many in the field believe that maladies like chronic fatigue syndrome and fibromyalgia directly result from an overstressed lifestyle, and that countless other health conditions are exacerbated or become chronic because of an impaired immune response" (p. 135).

According to McGraw (2001) the positive and negatives that an individual fixates on and internalizes; the self-praise or criticism; the distorted views of the world and themselves are all expressed in internal dialogue. Internal dialogue is the real-time conversation that one has with one's self about everything that is going on in their life. It encompasses all of self-talk, whether positive and rational or self-destructive and negative. McGraw believes that internal dialogue is constant and triggers a physiological change. Thus, if internal dialogue is pessimistic and defeatist it can be as destructive to physical health as any injury or virus. If it is really active, it can become so loud and pervasive that one fails to see important messages from others.

Rationally optimistic thoughts may be pushed aside because negative internal dialogue gets the loudest when one needs it the least. It gets the loudest when the pressure is on, because it flows at least in part from personal truth. When one is mentally and emotionally at war with one's self, it changes their physiology. It is also possible for internal dialogues to be quite rational and productive. Thinking rational, positive, and empowering thoughts results in each cell in the body responding with more positive and empowering energy. Positive internal dialogue consists of thoughts, messages, and fact-based rhetoric that allow one to live in accordance with reality (McGraw, 2001).

There are many other methods that work as well. Louise Hay (2000) explains that your mind is a tool for you to use in any way you wish. The way one now uses their mind is only a habit, and habits can be changed. The thoughts one "chooses" to think create the experiences they have. If an individual believes that it is hard or difficult to change a habit or a thought, then the choice of this thought will make it true for them. But, if one chooses to think it is becoming easier for me to make changes, then the choice of this thought will make that true for them. Identifying negative automatic reactions that may be unrealistic, irrational or distorted thoughts, is important.

The Wellness Book offers a comprehensive approach to breaking these negative automatic reactive habits. Cognitive restructuring does not gloss over or deny negative feelings or distress, but emphasizes paying attention to how thoughts influence feelings in order to avoid excessive emotions. So that these emotions are not the only way one feels. When governed by strong emotions, the mind becomes a filter, letting into consciousness only those thoughts that reinforce that mood, and little else is let through (Bensen & Stuart, 1993).

Many of the women in this study went through some phase of depression and then at some point acceptance. They then focused on the fact that: I have this condition, I have had it for some time, I have not been living my life as I want to, now what do I have to do to get back into life?

Often, it was financial concerns of the participants that controlled their progress. Going to doctors, having tests, experimenting with medications and alternative therapies, and missing work became expensive. In some cases it was the fear of being bedridden, or never becoming an active person again involved in participating in many activities life.

According to Rubenfeld (1997) people store their memories and emotional reactions to their life experiences in their bodies in ways that they are not usually aware of. By giving the impression that all is well, in spite of an experience having been toxic or traumatic, these feelings and the stress still show up in their bodies.

Humans have survival mechanisms that can roughly be divided into two functional categories: growth and protection. Protection is essential for survival, and growth is constant as every day billions of cells in the body wear out and need to be replaced.

But these are opposing survival mechanisms. The mechanisms that support growth and protection cannot operate optimally at the same time. Cells cannot simultaneously move forward and backward. Humans unavoidably restrict their growth behaviors when they shift into a protective mode. An individual can survive while under stress from perceived threats but chronic inhibition of growth mechanisms severely compromises their vitality.

It is also important to note that to fully experience vitality it takes more than just getting rid of life's stressors. In a growth/protection continuum, eliminating the stressors only puts one at the neutral point in the range. To fully thrive, an individual must eliminate the stressors and also actively seek joyful, loving, fulfilling lives that stimulate growth processes.

In response to perceived stress, hormones and chemicals are produced and secreted which prepare the body for the fight or flight response but inhibits growth processes and compromises the body's survival by interfering with the generation of vital energy reserves. When the body is mobilized for fight or flight response, the adrenal hormones directly repress the action of the immune system to conserve energy reserves, and interfere with one's ability to fight disease (Rubenfeld, 1997).

Almost every major illness that people acquire has been linked to chronic stress (Kopp & Rethelyi, 2004; McEwen & Lasley, 2002; McEwen & Seeman, 1999. Segerstrom & Miller, 2004). It becomes important therefore, to examine how an individual's fears and the ensuing protection behaviors impact their lives. What fears are stunting their growth, where did these fears come from? Are they necessary, or real? Are they contributing to a full life? If one can control one's fears, they can regain control over their lives, and letting go of their fears is the first step toward creating a fuller, more satisfying life.

And, why do I believe these women achieved a degree of better health? Because they wanted to, they developed a healing attitude, so they tried more things to help them to be well. One woman told me that "I tried so many no's I'm now on my way to yes." A concern for several of the women was that they are getting older and are running out of time, so they have to try harder. They asked themselves the question: Do I want the rest of my life to be sick or to be well? Or they stated that "I want the quality of my life to be better."

Jahnke (1999) states that if one has internally agreed to make choices that equate with joy, satisfaction, and trust, then a positive physiological response occurs throughout the body, particularly in the immune system. In the past this was called positive thinking or mental healing. Most experts in the field of mind-body medicine and healing agree both meditation and prayer are forms of focused intention. Both produce relaxation and shifts in brain-wave frequency and body chemistry.

A lot of recent research has supported the role of prayer in the healing process. When one triggers the healing system with self-applied health enhancement methods and then also triggers the power of the belief system, the capacity for heightened human potential and for recovery from disease is greatly magnified. From ancient time through the present, the most revered healers have known that the human being has a vital self-healing capacity that is profoundly influenced by faith and emotional harmony. Soon self-healing will become as common as aspirin and antibiotics have been in the past (Jahnke, 1999).

*"It is such a relief when you first find out that the
pain really does have a name,
and then you will ask (and everyone does), just where
can I place all the blame?
But even with knowing the best, the worst, all the
pitfalls the future could hold,
You still have a choice, you quit or fight,
you determine the story that's told."*
- *Rita Shaw*

Chapter 7. Introducing the Ladies

Blossom   Age: 64

Whatever I said I was going to do, you could go away, it would get done? Then I started getting unreliable. Instead of being ten minutes early, I was ten minutes late. Instead of following through on some assignment, I would have to call someone and tell them I wasn't going to be able to finish it.

And it was stressful, phantom pains started, bouts of crying like I was pregnant, bouts of diarrhea for no reason. Doctors, ran tests for various things, they couldn't find anything. But I felt fatigued, and I didn't know why I was so tired. They said it was because of the stress. It was the same stress level that I always had. The more the doctors ran tests for other things, the more they said, here: take these mood altering drugs, you're depressed. Those pills of course, made me sick. But the more I said no, these pills are making me sick, I can't take these, the more they decided I needed some additional help. I need to see a therapist for mental illness.

I said: I'm not depressed, and you're not helping me". And one doctor told me I needed to get over that. Take these drugs, and I got referred to a psychiatrist too. The psychiatrist said, well, the only reason you need to see me if you want me to give you some drugs. Well, I didn't need drugs; I needed to find out what was wrong. Muscle aches, joint aches, it might be there for an hour, or a month. I thought I needed a hip replacement. It was the fibromyalgia. I had bumped my knees, and I thought I had really done some damage to my knee, it was the fibromyalgia. The more they run tests and scratch their head, the more they're telling me that I'm depressed. Well now I'm starting to get depressed.

I knew something was wrong with me. The doctors kept telling me nothing is wrong, it's all in my mind, it's all in my head. At the time fibromyalgia was not known as a disease. This was maybe ten years ago. And it became recognized as a disease, but the doctors didn't recognize it. They just said: Oh, that's just something that they put a name to, to give you all something to say, but it's really all just in your head. So, now they have a named disease out there that doesn't exist. You're depressed and you're having some mental problems

But, they still want to get you a lot of mood altering medications. Some of the mood altering medications will make you hurt yourself. If only they would tell you what it was going to do. I was at the stove, I had the pot in one hand and I dropped something off the cooking fork into the fire. And I reached my bare hand in the fire. I ended up dropping the pot, and almost scalded myself when I realized what I was doing. That's just one example.

I read a lot. I had gotten into part of this story that I just wanted to know what was going to happen next. On the way home from work, I was driving down interstate 80; there was no traffic ahead of me. I keep thinking about this book, it started taking precedence. I mean it was compulsion. I just had to know what happened next. And I kept turning around in the seat trying to reach this book. I'm still driving 80 mph. I'm watching the traffic, and there's no car immediately near me. I forced myself to keep driving and not reach back there. And then suddenly I couldn't stand it anymore and I practically turned around, got the bag, got it close to me. Pulled the book out, turned back around, propped the book up on the steering wheel and started reading. No idea that I was driving still, no idea that I was on the expressway. A car a couple of blocks ahead of me changed lanes, and that shift got my attention.

To prescribe that for me. I told the doctor I couldn't take those, they make me sick. He said OK, what do they do? And I told him. He tore the prescription up. And said oh, no.

I'm not supposed to be lifting heavy things. We had to change from cast iron skillets, and those things. Taking the garbage out is a problem. You can't let the garbage get too full, because that might be the day you can't lift it. My life is in my purse; I can't carry that around. Don't travel, unless you have somebody to handle your luggage. Putting it in the car, taking it out of the car.

It was my rheumatologist who first diagnosed me. He was pressing on these little things. And it didn't hurt when he touched them. It hurt immediately afterwards. It was like delayed reaction. On some of those points, no matter how lightly, I got either a burning sensation or some other sensation. I was very sore when he got through because now he woke up all these spots all over my body.

And it's probably due to fibromyalgia setting in, it's in my ears. That's a problem, so my ears keep filling with fluid. But with the pains deep set in my ears, by the eardrum, or whatever, I'm not getting the response that I should be getting, and I'm losing total sensation of up/down.

You have basically 24-hour pain, some part of your body hurts all the time. And I don't take the pain medications. I refuse to take something. Mine settles in my bones also, not just the muscles. But you do what you got do. I don't know what else to tell you.

Once I got diagnosed, there was relief, immediately. No one was trying to pressure me to be depressed anymore. Though they were still trying to get me to take medication for the problem. But I don't want my body building up the tolerance for the pain relievers. It starts tightening up, and once its starts tightening up, the fibromyalgia kicks in likes it's a live person, and says oh goody, let's jump in there and help be stressful.

So, I finally came to a halt and I was body scanning. And I had a surprised look, and felt surprised. So I body scanned again. What was wrong was that nothing hurt! And that was so funny, once I figured out what it was. In that particular moment, nothing hurt. Fingernails didn't hurt, hair didn't hurt, nose didn't hurt, eyes, legs, knees – nothing hurt. I was on a cruise. I was away from work, away from everybody else. I just assumed it was just being away from everything. Being away from the stress.

I stopped worrying about anyone else, and it released me, helped me to go rest when I needed to. Not responding to other people's needs. I'll ride with someone, but I won't drive. If I didn't feel like getting plane tickets, I decided I didn't want to be there. The thing that I've been fighting right now is taking naps, I've just decided that I'm just going to go ahead and I'm not going fight it. Just let the body slow down, let everything come down to a lower pace.

Some of the other things about being better. I can travel; I can do short bursts of things, ordinary things. You know, I can get it to the stove, leave it on the stove until you can take it off. It makes the house messier, yes, and housework, let it go. If you feel like doing it, do it. If not, and nobody else does it, let it stay there. The house won't burn down from it. I'll still have a roof over my head. Just walk around the mess. Hour by hour, day by day, week, by week; and after a while you start breathing better. And guess what – it didn't disintegrate, everything was fine. It makes it little more messy, but it's livable. And again, once you get past the guilt.

Dahlia   Age: 65

I used to be able to do pretty much what I wanted. I'd walk all the time. In fact, I did a 17-mile hike up a mountain and down. Now I'm lucky I can get in and out of a car. I'm very limited to what I can do. I take a lot of pain medications, and it really helps me to be able to do things. And sometimes I'll do things and I know I'm going to be miserable, but I just tell myself: "This too shall pass", and in a few days it does. People that see me and know me say they can't believe that I have these limitations. In fact, I have a cane, but I don't use it around people that I know because I don't want them to know about it.

I went to the doctor and I said: "just everything hurts me, to touch me hurts me". So he sent me to a pain specialist, and that woman like saved my life. It was wonderful. She said: "You have fibromyalgia". She put me on the Elavil to sleep at night, and it was like I died and went to heaven. I hadn't felt that good in a long time, I was able to sleep. I can't do a lot of the things that I used to be able to do. And some days, I don't really know what triggers it. You know, some days you feel good, some days you don't feel good. And, I'm in love with my heating pad it really helps. I have a lot of trouble sleeping at night. I found out about the fibromyalgia when I went to my doctor and I complained to him about everything that hurt. He would poke me and I would scream and practically leap out of the chair, and I thought what in the world? And for a long time that bothered me, that nobody knew what it was. But I wake up every hour or two during the night because this shoulder hurts on the left, so I'll turn over and sleep on the right side for a while. I'll flip flop all night long.

As long as I can function, I know my limitations. But right now my fibromyalgia, it's kinda leveled off. I not a hero, I'm not a martyr or anything, but you know, you can't give in to this stuff. The more you give into it, the less you'll be able to do. So, I just keep moving along. It's difficult. I'm up early and I keep busy all day doing different things. And I sit down in front of the TV at night, and I'm really, really tired at the end of the day. And I believe that when you have a lot of pain and stuff, you just keep trying to go along with it and hang in there.

Like I explained, I have quite a few health problems, and I've always got one crisis after another, you know, pick a part of the body. And, I just have sorta gotten to the point where I just kinda of ignore things. And when new things come up, like I had all this dizziness and I had to go to an ear specialist. So she said she thought I has a brain tumor. So she sent me to for tests. My husband asked: "Are you upset?" And I said: "I am just so aggravated." I just get aggravated.

And like I said, I don't even tell people half of the time. I don't care to talk about it. Because I've had these problems for so long. I think I've had fibromyalgia for a very long time, and I know it's hard to diagnose, and not all doctors are in agreement that it exists. Because of all of my problems, I have learned to just ignore it all, believe it or not. And if things hurt, I just kinda cuss under by breath and just keep on moving. Basically, it's what I do.

If and when I'm free of it, I'll probably have a ticker tape parade for myself. You know you go along, and you hope you're going to get better, and what have you. But, like I said before, I have my good days, and my bad days. But my family is very protective of me, and I don't like it at all. I want them, to treat me like a normal person and I tell them if it hurts, I'll stop and sit down. So let's not make an issue out of it. I don't even think that everybody knows that I have fibromyalgia.

I believe that my health problems were due to being married to an abusive man and being in constant tension and what have you. He actually tried to kill me. But, he got sick and died, so, I didn't have to finish with the divorce. I've been listening and reading about it and I believe that's been a very large and contributing factor.

I read about this condition or problem because, you know, I'd like to know what they're doing for it 'cause it doesn't seem to get an awful lot of attention. And I would love to be in a support group with people because sometimes you meet people that have a problem and you can say: "you know, I read in so-and-so, that this-and-that." And you can tell them and it will help people. I know the same medication or the same exercise is not going to help everybody, but you just never know.

Daisy   Age: 65

Before I had joint and body pain, I didn't have any physical limitations. Only age related or other medical conditions. Now, the amount of activity – physical activity my body can handle is limited. I run a boarding house, and I keep up the boarding house. It consists of a lot of work. Many of these things, since rheumatoid arthritis hit me, I have to either hire someone or get help from one of my adult children.

My pain killer regime allows me to be more physical than I could be without it. It's a fairly heavy pain regime. I use a transdermal patch. The patch is changed every 72 hours. I get break-through pain, but I can handle that. The patch works fairly well. That enables me to maximize what my body can do. However, with or without narcotics or pain medications, fibromyalgia or rheumatoid arthritis still limits what I can do, because my hands and wrists, hips and feet are affected most by it. So I sometimes I need a cane. Sometimes my wrists and hands are basically incapable of doing much of anything when they get quite inflamed.

The disease presented itself first as rheumatoid arthritis. I spent about a year in a wheelchair. It came on rather quickly. I thought I was coming down with a virus. And then within a day, all of sudden, most of my joints and muscles, joints actually, I couldn't support my own weight, dress myself. And my internist sent me to a rheumatologist. And said you are flaring up with rheumatoid arthritis. He did tests; I was on a steroid regime for about 8 months. Then we had to come to a decision. I had come down in dosage to a fairly lower dose, but it still was affecting the other medical conditions that I have, and my internist decided that we would just have discontinue everything.

My muscles remained really quite strong and I was able to do a lot of walking before this hit. My lifestyle change is that I have to space the amount of time I use my muscles. That's how the fibromyalgia is presenting itself now, 5 years after the original flare-up of rheumatoid arthritis. So, how I handle it is daily. By spacing my activities, I'll be active for perhaps a half an hour, sit, watch television, or read for half-hour.

Things seem to equalize themselves. I don't know that I live much differently than a lot of people that are around 65, men or women. Mostly by this time in life, you get a few chronic conditions. So I have to say I don't think I would be doing things much differently. I would not have as many limits on what I can physically do in one stretch at a time. I tire easily, even after half an hour of say, walking or something of that sort. Because, I'm an older person, most everyone my age is not doing a heck of lot more.

I would like to be disease free. How it would affect me the most is I wouldn't have to depend on pain medication and that in itself, has side effects that go with it. And I probably think the biggest thing would be that I wouldn't have to use narcotics. Which adds to being older. In the fact, that I have to be extra careful with doing physical things. And then your memory isn't always at it best when you're 65. And narcotics sure don't help.

If you were used to a high activity lifestyle, I think it would affect you more, and you would have a harder time adjusting. But, the stimulus of wanting to remain more active, might in itself, act as placebo towards the illness.

I used to travel a great deal. And I found that I don't have a great desire to travel, because for some reason I like being closer to home. The only place I'd ever move to, would be the bottom of a hill of an emergency room. And I guess when we get older, that's kinda how we feel. We want to have closer contact with medical help. And, the fibromyalgia has given me an attitude where I'm not a gamy about doing things, and traveling is one of them, as I was before this condition.

Flora   Age: 63

I worked, 30 hours a week. I also did volunteer work through the church. My regular doctor asked me to go to a specialist for my thyroid; I was having a lot of pain in my throat. He said I want you to see a rheumatologist, because I hurt. My throat hurt me and around my whole neck hurt me; I had lots of aches and pains. He knew I had arthritis. I went to the rheumatologist and she immediately said I had 14 tender spots. It was a relief, because I thought I had cancer. I had so much pain in and around my neck and my throat that nothing in this world except cancer would give such pain, such constant pain. So it was a relief when I found out I had fibromyalgia. I was not happy, it got to the point where I couldn't get up from a chair without being in pain and holding on to the table. 'Cause I have said, I don't want to live. There was no suicide or anything. I prayed and I said: "Lord, if I have to live like this, I would rather die. Show me a way to help myself, or the doctors to help me, or take me because I can't live like this". And I was only in my early 50's at the time.

My rheumatologist said I needed to sleep better, so we were experimenting with the different antidepressants. She did tell me about the different types of exercises I should be doing. They helped me to a point. But I wasn't satisfied, so I started buying all these different books on exercise. From tai chi, yoga, and massage therapy – I tried all of them. And I found the best, especially for my arms, is isometrics. I have been to an osteopath, and I was told that I had chronic tendentious. Which, the funniest thing is, since I've been doing the isometrics, I'm not having the elbow pain like I used to. I do use the heat patches, which help a lot 'cause sometimes the pain won't go away no matter what, so I do the heat patches for about 2 days straight and it will go away, I'll heal.

Now my life is a complete turnaround! I no longer do any volunteer work. When I do my housework, I will wash 1/3 of the kitchen floor, and then I'll rest, and then another third, and another third, until I finish it. When I do go out with my friends I don't do anything the day before and the day after. Fatigue is my worst enemy. I still can't control that. And if I do push myself – I'm bad for the next 2 days. I will cook a large meal once or twice a week, and then put some in the freezer. The cleaning up is the worst. By the time you cook and you eat, you don't want to clean up. I've gone into using paper plates, even plastic silverware. I do a lot of vitamins and supplements. And there are several things I've learned from the books on fibromyalgia. You do need the different supplements. So, that's how I work it out. My mental state, God takes care of that. I mean, He showed me these books. He inspired me to do all that. I also feel good, I always have been a real good, happy person. And I like sharing with other people that's why I joined the arthritis group. That just keeps me going, caring for other people that helps make me happy. You need to accept it, and not let it take over. You need to take control and not let it get you down. You take your life and you say what's important. And you say, ok, if I don't do this, I'm going to end up the way that I used to be. And I don't want that.

Now, they've said that trauma sometimes goes along with the fibromyalgia. I've been to many groups. And people said they were in car accident, one was abused. I'm just wondering, I don't remember much about my childhood. My mother, when she was carrying my brother, she said she sang the whole time. When she was carrying me, 2 years later, she was always walking around with a black eye. My father abused her. My mother said she cried during her whole pregnancy with me. And I'm thinking, could this be something? Also, my brother, who is 2 years older, thought I was a toy, and he tried to break me. My brother tied me up to the table leg and he threw darts at my back. He shot rubber bands at me, he punched me. My terrible temper. I think it was because my mother and father were divorced. So I'm' just wondering whether it was me being in my mother's womb and her crying all the time. Or my brother picking on me, and kinda beating me up. Not beating me to the point where I had black and blue marks, just enough.

Of course I want to be well. But, I don't believe I ever will be. And that's why I have to keep it under control. I can't let it get to me. You know, there's rheumatologist is doing research with blood tests. Well, maybe in 20 years, she'll find something. But, I really don't think so and I can't wait that long. I'm 63 years old, and so I know I just have to take what I can. There's so much I want to go back to, traveling and helping more than I do. But I know it's impossible. So I just have to accept my life as it is.

You need a very good support group. That's very important. You need people who have the problem. Even like when I was younger, I was anemic, and I would go with one of my friends and I would say: "I'm tired." And she told me she couldn't understand why I was so tired. How I could be tired. In fact, this guy and I broke up because he couldn't stand me always saying I'm tired.

I just want to repeat you have to take control. Doctors only tell you 50%. The other 50% you have to learn. You have to know your options, what to do. You have to use yourself as a guinea pig.

Heather   Age: 56

I do everything now, that I did before, but not as well, and I have really bad days of pain and then I'm really grouchy. I guess I slept better and was less grouchy. I can't remember because pain has become pretty much a daily thing, and so you learn to live with it, and you kind of get desensitized to it. So you try different things. I've had fibromyalgia less than 5 years, I can't remember exactly when I started having serious problems with it, or when I was diagnosed with it.

I had several things wrong with me at the same time so part of that could have been because of the fibromyalgia going somewhere else. At the time I was diagnosed, I was referred to a specialist, a rheumatologist, because my primary care physician felt that I might have rheumatoid arthritis. He did some testing and decided that, that was not the case, fortunately. I had osteoarthritis, golfers elbow, tendonitis of the right thumb, and something in the right trapezious area. I received injections in the socket of my right wrist. I received an injection in the trapezious at that time as well. Very painful shots. I didn't think I could hurt more than I did. Almost passed out, had to lie down for quite a while before I returned to whatever normal is, and could sit up again. It takes a while for the shots to kick in, and there was some improvement after the injections. I ended up, especially in the trapezious area, it was able to go down the arm and so it kind of took care of the shoulder area and the elbow. He also thought I had reverse carpal tunnel, which I had never heard of, because I've already had carpal tunnel surgery.

So, on good days I'm in pain, and on bad days I'm in a lot of pain. And it doesn't necessarily stop me from doing what I was doing, like going to Great America. But, instead of walking I will rent a cart and ride it. Because I also have trouble with the hip area. It's either related to the osteoarthritis, or you know. Regardless of what it's related to, it hurts, so I ride. You're going to be in pain, OK. If I'm going to hurt, whether I'm doing something or not, then I might as well do something and have fun. So, I didn't let it stop me.

I've tried outer healing things, like copper magnets, and strong magnets. In fact, I'm wearing a magnet bracelet now. It's not so much that it gets rid of the pain, but when I take them off and don't wear them for a couple of days, I feel it. And, I'm hoping this summer to be down to only wearing it at night and not during the day 'cause I don't want a tan line. Well, see I just take it nonchalantly, that's life, deal with it.

Spiritually, I have strong faith, and I believe that God walks with me in everything. And I can do all things through He who strengthens me. So, I continue to do. It's an action verb. If I were free from it, I would be in less pain. And I would sleep better every night. I don't let it keep me from doing things as long as I can get up and go. Sometimes it keeps me from going on certain water slides because of the stairs that you have to climb. But it didn't stop me from para-sailing or bunging jumping last summer.

So, I'm not sure I let it totally interfere with what I'm doing. I might have to limit the extent of what I do, but as far as doing things, now that I have somebody to do stuff with, I do it. And, so I don't really know how life would be different. I never really thought about being free of it. It's so... I just have goals in life and one of my goals in life is to make somebody laugh every day. Laughter is healing mechanism. I feel if I'm sick or something, I haven't been laughing enough. So, I try to laugh more. But I have a saying: if I had fun, I won. And so, when you kind of live with that kind of perspective, you find the humor and the fun on all situations. Not to say that I don't get down and out from time to time, but usually when things are going bad eventually I just stop and I think of how much worse they could have been. I mean, I'm not a total Pollyanna, but I think about other people who have to live through so much worse stuff, from my perspective, that I try and count my blessings.

And, have an attitude of gratitude. Because there are people without limbs, there are people who are deaf, blind, have lost everything in a fire, or tornado, or flood. I'm very blessed. And, in all things give thanks. You know, scripture. It kinda tells me what I need to do. It doesn't always work – so I say: God help me. I'm a mental health therapist; I work for a mental health agency. With the pain, sometimes I am in tears. I'm not glossing this over. Sometimes I have shooting pain that is just unbearable. So, sometimes it limits me. But I try not to let it because life's short.

    I think that part of the reason why I have the attitude that I have is because I have lost most of the people in my life that are important to me. I've lost all grandparents, and aunts, uncles, parents and a sister. I've lost a best friend through death. And when you go through that kind of thing, when they die suddenly its one kind of grieving. When they die over a period of time it's a totally different set of grieving and you just realize how short life is, and you decide to either get what you can out of life or always wishing coulda, shoulda, woulda. I have very few regrets in choices, big choices that I made. You know, we always do stupid little things, and oh, I wish I wouldn't have done that. But I think that that changes your perspective on life in general. Also, I think that part of what has kept me out of the normal pity party is that you can only feel sorry for yourself for so long and then you run out of material. I think that what's kept me moving and functioning and not being depressed is that I'm on medication. I take quite a bit of medication.

    Sometimes, you're like: I'm never going to be thankful for this. And then you know, you realize what you learned from that experience, and how you've grown and changed because of it. And what level of interaction and interpersonal skills you can have with other people. Because of being there, and knowing something about some of what they are experiencing.

The antidepressant and mood stabilizing that I was taking I was prescribed about 2 years prior to my fibromyalgia onset. And so, I think it helped me deal with the symptoms, but they were not prescribed for it. A significant amount of time that it didn't really affect one way or the other. Other than because I'm stabilized and functioning very well, it helps you know it just all fits in with that. Some people can have what I had mental health wise and be on disability and not function. I'm a little bit too stubborn for that. And again, it goes back to having fun. And so, you know, that's just kind of how it is.

Hyacinth   Age: 54

I do everything. I do housework, I do yard work, physically I do anything that I want to do. I have to be careful about how I lift or how long I work, and I have to sit down sometimes and just rest, or take a break, and then I'm good to go, but I really don't have a limit on what I do.

I was going to my chiropractor for years with pain in my hip for scoliosis and my shoulder, but that seemed to have intensified, and so I was going to her more and more and wasn't getting better. I was going for massage therapy as well, I was doing both and didn't get the kind of relief that I wanted.

I went to a general practitioner, and I had a whole list of things and he stopped me at three. We had enough to deal with, three items. I remember him giving me some kind of medication, I don't remember what is was, I didn't take it for more than maybe 2 weeks, because I didn't like it, it bothered my stomach. From there I did get diagnosed by a psychiatrist, nobody seemed to know what I had, it was confusing everybody, and I felt like I was going kinda whacky. Nobody seemed to understand what I was talking about.

I found this book at the bookstore that had a picture on the cover, and it showed the points that were bilateral on the different parts of the body that I recognized that was the pattern that I felt. I took that to my GP, and said: "well, here's what I think I have". I just felt like I needed a positive diagnosis. I didn't know what that was going to do for me, I was hoping that there would be some relief I would get from the diagnosis. He did some checking, and he said, yes, you definitely have fibromyalgia. His suggestion was probably medication, because I think neurologically there is some connection with messing up your sleep pattern or something. So he wasn't terribly helpful to me. I was still miserable.

I went to see a Chinese doctor and he explained to me that fibromyalgia was called 'traveling pain'. Because there were times when I would feel it in different parts of my body, it wasn't the same place all the time. And he said they were treating that for thousands of years in China, and he said that he could help me. I trusted what he had to say, I liked him, I thought he was sincere, and I figured what have I got to lose? You know Chinese medicine has been around for centuries. So I trusted him, and he has seen me through this and that's basically what helped me the most. It was acupuncture, but also Chinese herbs that I would take for my aches and pains.

I knew that I had to make lifestyle changes, and I knew that I had to help myself. I think part of it is personality, I have a kind of tenacity, if I want to do something, I'm going to do it. And I'm willing to put the time and effort into it. And I think that and my faith has seen me through. That's basically what I attribute to my success so far.

My doctor encouraged me to find ways of helping myself. My chiropractor is wonderful, she gives me her opinion, and I respect her for that. And I think I gained more confidence in what I was doing just by having other people, who I respect in the medical field, validate what I was doing. And I think that was a big help. My Chinese doctor, I felt he was sincere as well, he was trying very hard to make me feel better. So I think I was surrounded by good medical people. It kind of encouraged me to keep trying, that I would feel better someday. I never thought I would feel this good though, and that's the truth.

Right now I don't feel like I am suffering from it pretty much at all. I have morning stiffness, but I talk to other people my age and I don't think it's a lot different than what I feel. My sleep pattern is much improved. Occasionally I have this sleeplessness, but not like before. And I really don't think of fibromyalgia anymore. It used to occupy my thoughts. I think that a real turning point for me was when I went to the class at the hospital, and I saw other people who had fibromyalgia. Most of them were females; most of them looked horrible. Some of them had quit their jobs and succumbed to the disease, and I said no, that's not going to be me. I think that maybe that was a motivating factor for me, that I didn't want to be one of *them*. So, it was a big struggle, but getting up in the morning without feeling like I'm ninety-five, however that's supposed to feel like, is a blessing to me. There are still days when I get up and I am limping along for an hour or so, but it's not like before, where I could barely get out of bed. And I would be so tired I could hardly function. I don't have that anymore.

I have things to do, and places to go, and that too was my motivator. I don't have that kind of pain any more. Right now I have found a way to kind of use my acupuncture, my chiropractor and my doctor and my personal trainer, to mold me into a sense of well-being. To where I can exercise 3 times a week and not suffer terribly. And there were times that I thought that being a cripple and being a nonfunctioning member of society was a reality. And I said no I can't do this. I think that the biggest thing I have done, lifestyle change, is work my way into exercising again. I know that's a real key into feeling good. And having a sense of well-being and saying healthy.

I was diagnosed with fibromyalgia in I think 1998. I remember going to an exercise class and my recovery time was unbelievable. I was so stiff from doing aerobics; I was only 28 at the time. My recovery time should not have been that long. It had to be least a week where I could barely get out of a chair. I was just like an old person, hobbling around. And I really didn't think that the exercises were all that strenuous. But it did pass. But I do think about that, that something wasn't right. But I had other things going on in my life. I was trying to have a baby; I didn't have time for that stuff.

Having talked to other people with fibromyalgia, I know sometimes there is an activating event that brings it on. In 1993, I took a very bad fall and I broke my ankle in two places, and dislocated it. And I was home for 6 months. But they say that sometimes that happens, that you suffer the effects of fibromyalgia after something traumatic like an operation. I did have surgery; I had surgery that very morning. And it was very big deal in my life, and I didn't like it.

Another thing I think, I'm not sure about this either, but in 1998, I was probably perimenapausal. Every month I would suffer with the chills. I remember sitting in the air-conditioned family room, with flannel pajamas on, and 2 blankets, and a hat on my head watching TV in the rocking chair. That was the only chair I would be fairly comfortable in. When I think back, it may have just been all individual medical things going on with me, there could be a connection.

I began feeling better when I started to going to my acupuncture doctor. I knew that there was help for me, and it came in the form of a little Chinese man! And all his herbs and treatment. I would say it took maybe 6 months of intensive treatment with I'm before I started feeling like I could get my life back. He didn't go after the fibromyalgia from the start; he went after the sleep pattern. He said first you treat the acute condition, then you treat the chronic. Because the pain was keeping me awake. If he could treat the sleep pattern I could get my restorative sleep hours, that would help my chronic condition, and that's how I got better.

Well, I would say – don't give up. I would say try every possible means of treatment. Unconventional medicine seems to be what worked for me. Read as much as you can, get as much information as possible. And talk to other people who have it. What worked for me may not work for somebody else. I also happened on an excellent personal trainer who listened. Again, find people who will listen to you. But I think you also have to be somewhat informed, so you ask the right questions, and I think you have to take a personal responsibility in your care, and what is happening to you. And if you don't like something, you have to speak up.

I had lots of things going on with my family. The death of my sister, mother and father, all within a couple of years. But even through those very stressful times, the worst of the fibromyalgia had passed. I still went to my acupuncture doctor, but I would say it was very much under control at that time. Because it would have been impossible. Unbelievable those were extremely stressful times. I had my flare ups, but I never had my bad, bad symptoms of fibromyalgia, because it was under control.

From the way I understand it from my Chinese doctor, your body is out of balance, you have too much acid, too much of something. What his job is, is to balance this out, internally. That's apparently what he did because I am feeling a whole lot better. So my advice is try acupuncture.

Iris   Age: 55

Prior to fibromyalgia, I could walk about 3 miles twice a day. I could play tennis for a couple of hours every day. I could get a good night's sleep, wake up refreshed, and could get through the day. Without wanting to take a nap, without wanting to lay down after washing the dishes, without wanting to lay down after doing the laundry. Not having to want to lie down after cleaning up or vacuuming the house. With fibromyalgia, I feel as though I have more limited expanses of expendable energy.

I also had other childhood diseases, such as scarlet fever, and measles. I had mumps in high school, I'm not sure if any of those other childhood diseases also contributed, somehow I feel that my immune system has been compromised. I was diagnosed with fibromyalgia a couple of years ago. I had gone to a napropath and a cardiologist office, after experiencing what I thought was chest pains. All of the tests were negative for any type of cardio involvement. The doctor was basically baffled by the pain in my heart and in my chest. And he was the first person to ever suggest that it was possible I had a fibromyalgia pain that was moving to different parts of my body, which included my heart. Which was something very new to me, I never heard that, although I was trying to read about fibromyalgia, that it could move to different parts of your body, and affect different parts of your body at different times.

So basically, what I have been doing for the last 18 years – is going from doctor to doctor trying to find out what is wrong with me. And until recently, there wasn't even a name for anything that was wrong with me. I also might have chronic fatigue syndrome, which is not helping either. And I think that somehow they are related also. I personally think that I have some type of a viral invasion in my body, and that this invasion has affected my muscles. In addition to that, my doctor had suggested that he thought that maybe I was depressed. So, he sent me to a psychiatrist and I can't tell you the name of all the so-called psychiatric medications for either depression or anxiety that they tried on me. That absolutely gave me no relief; I had more problems with the side effects of every single medication that they put me on. From blurred vision, to palpitations, to stomach pain, to increased insomnia. So, none of those types of treatments were of any value to me.

At one point, time, I would say about 5 or 6 years, ago, my doctor then decided to try to put me on prednisone, which he did. And I was on it for maybe 3 months, which was a little bit too long. I felt very good and I had more energy.

I think it somehow became toxic in my body because I build up the medication in different particles of the food that are breaking down, that don't get out of my body fast enough, and therefore rather than helping me it becomes toxic. Rather than my food giving me more energy, it sits in body and becomes basically rotted out and toxic. So, I think, that I'm not healthy because my system inside is not functioning completely. And it's breaking down and fighting against myself. I don't sleep well at night. I'm still looking for treatments. So far, the things that have worked the best for me is to get outside for 15 to 20 minutes in the sunshine every day. One of the things that has helped me the best, is to have massages. Now that I'm having more frequent massages, it does seem to help with the pain and to move around. My lymph system does not remove toxins adequately. So having head to toe massages, at least twice a month, has been one of the few things that has helped me to feel a little bit better, I can get a little bit of relief from pain.

I went to a chiropractor and I also had acupuncture done on me. The acupuncture actually hurt worse when they were putting the needles in. And they could not believe how much pain I had just by them putting the needles in. And I got no relief, I had no increased energy, I had no results, and I wanted to have results. Or that I had resistance. Maybe, up to 10 treatments. And to me it was a waste of money. And really painful, it was a painful treatment.

It was suggested to me that I do colonics, and I tried to do that route. And I had one colonic and I thought I would go through the roof. It was extremely painful. I had also tried the steam. You get into a steam tent and try to detoxify yourself with a wrap – a special wrap of chemicals and herbs. I tried this high heat detoxification and that really didn't get me any good results. Also, there's footbath that you put your feet in – electronically or molecularly draws out the toxins.

And I tried that foot treatment bath a couple of times. I don't know if I don't do enough of the treatments to give me the results that they want. Or if I'm just too discouraged that I don't get any results or any relief that I don't think it's worth my money. Saunas seem to help me. And I feel better with a dry sauna type of heat, than anything else. So I would say, bufferin, massage and a sauna so far are the only 3 things that basically help me or make me feel comfortable, to where my pain isn't excruciating. I have different levels of pain, it's not always intense, it's not always high levels of pain. It varies from day to day and from activity to activity as far as how much pain I have or how much pain I don't have. But is a constant every day, never go away pain. It something I live with, it's something I try to ignore.

And in fact, I have been trying to read books on healing myself and listening to tapes. I went to a lecture, and it was very interesting, as the point of it was that you are either making yourself healthy or ill at a cellular level depending on what your mind is saying to your body. And I think that was the thing that made the most sense to me and has helped me the most. More than anything else, that I have heard or have tried to do, was that on a cellular level I can make a difference in my own body, by what I think and what I tell myself. I have been trying to tell myself is that I am happy, I am healthy, and I am well. I am trying to through my own meditation and reading and research, trying to make my own self-well.

One of the books I have read which I found very helpful is by Catherine Ponder, The Dynamic Laws of Healing. She talks about different issues such as forgiveness and anger. I feel that I have been very, very angry all my life. I personally think this anger has turned inward, and that my cells have been reacting to a lifelong anger. I have not been successful in dealing with the anger, and I have not realized until recently how much the anger can hurt my body. And I feel that this is the source of my pain and illness along with the viruses that have attacked my body along the way. I believe that the combination of these two things from an emotional and mental side I am trying to control or somehow deal with my emotions so that they are not as damaging to my body. So I continue to look for treatments, I continue to try different things. It seems to me that I have been reading that people who have positive friends and positive influences in their life are healthier. So basically what I'm trying to find are people in my life to have fun with. That's the treatment that I think that I need.

As far as taking care of myself. I am just now starting to take care of myself, I always put other people first, and I always put myself last and therefore I did not take care of myself as much as I took care of other people. So I think it's time I took care of myself. But I do need some exercise and some activity every day. I do need to express or share or release emotions that are not healthy for me. I do need some type of pain medication a couple of times a week. Sometimes I ice myself; sometimes I use heat to help relieve the pain. I'm still looking for different types of treatment.

I would like to sleep all night and wake up with a feeling of renewed energy. I would like to be pain free. I would like to be able to do the activities of daily living without being worn out. I have to do more things that make me happy. Walking my dog makes me happy. So I need to walk my dog every day and make myself happy. I am trying to be just a happy person, instead of a crabby painful person. I would like to be a happy carefree, free of bondage, and the fibromyalgia is part of the bondage.

There is something else that I have tried. I would drive to this doctor's office once a month and he would put an IV solution into me, hyperallementation, which was a high dosage of vitamins, minerals and fluids. I seemed to have a good response to his hyperfusion directly into my blood. I would feel better for about a week to 10 days. And then I would notice that my energy level would start going down again. But I felt that this was a very expensive form of treatment. So, I went to this person for about 6 months and discontinued the treatment. When I discontinued the treatment, I did not have any lasting results. The effects of the hyperalimentation were gone. It was something that I needed to do, basically on a monthly basis it seems like for the rest of my life. It was too expensive for me, but I did feel better when it was infused directly into my bloodstream. A higher dosage of a higher concentration of vitamins, minerals, and fluids. That made me feel better.

Jasmine   Age: 58

Before my diagnosis, and before the symptoms appeared – I was the mother of three young boys, all born within 4 ½ years. That kept me busy. I was also married to someone with a handicap, a one-sided paralysis, due to a driving accident. And so I was the person in family who carried everything, moved all the furniture. So physically I had a lot of heavy burdens to carry. I stayed pretty active. In high school and my first couple years of college I'd been pretty active in sports also. I was a gymnast, rode a bike a lot, and danced.

A typical day in my life then was very little sleep. The nights were very short, and someone was always teething or sick or had trouble sleeping. So, I was very sleep deprived, and that really seemed to compound the problem. It got to where I was having more frequent colds and flu, and right along with the kids. I was sick every time they were sick. And that was unusual, I'd always been real healthy. I have bad knees, even in high school.

I probably had been exhibiting symptoms of fibromyalgia for 4 or 5 years before I got the diagnosis. I'd gotten to point where my muscles would ache so badly that if I climbed to the top of the stairs, I would be cramped, in terrible pain; I would have to rest for minute before I could complete to do anything. I couldn't put the laundry away. My energy level dropped quite a bit. My joints would ache, I ached all over. So, that started when I went to nursing school in my early 30's.

My doctor talked about fibromyalgia. He was able to attribute it to previous stress in my life and was very good about talking and encouraging me to watch what exacerbated the problem and to rest which is not always easy to do. He prescribed Soma, and occasionally with a bad exacerbation like Tylenol 3 or a Vicadin, hydrocordone. And, I would go for a manipulation probably once a week at least. And with that I was able to keep functioning. I do believe that he did say that there seemed to be a correlation between some of the viruses going around and the incidences of chronic fatigue and fibromyalgia. He kinda put those things together. So at least I felt legitimate, vindicated a little bit.

I have learned to ignore pain a lot and to not rest until I absolutely had no choice because I can't keep going. I tend to be an optimist, and I think a lot of time that has stood me in good stead. And I know many times that I can ignore things and go ahead and accomplish what I have to do. I've learned that that's only for a period of time and I have to pay the price for ignoring it too long. So, I've learned over the years to rest.

I feel very close to God, and I was raised with affirmations. I was raised with affirming my health. I was raised with affirming my relationship with God and all creation. I had a respiratory cardiac arrest 35 years ago. And died while having a C-section. And I was wide-awake, I had a spinal. So, I knew I was dying. I went through that whole experience and that has served to make this physical in a way less important for me. I just don't tend to get wrapped up in what's going on with me physically ''cause I look beyond that.

And I have had only one time in my life when I was just about ready to give up and that was with pain. Before my parathyroid surgery I was in so much pain and that coupled with fibromyalgia and myofascia syndrome was just - I don't think I could have gone on in my life feeling that way, you know, forever. So, I got a dog. I got a four-legged furry therapist. That's what I got.

But I've also seen the correlation between sleep and depression and physical illness. If I'm sleeping well and more relaxed than I have a tendency to be much improved. So I that's half the battle right there.

I have been on anti-inflammatories for 10 years, at least. I ended up getting up on Viox when they upped my dosage; I ended up with micro valve and bicuspid valve prolapse. And now I can't tolerate much in the way of a lot of cardiac arrhythmias and lot of arrhythmia problems. I used to throw PVC's, maybe 20 an hour but I stayed on the medication because I hurt so badly otherwise. But now I take aspirin or one of the back and body medications. And that gives me some relief.

I had rotator cuff surgery. I fell. My balance isn't very good anymore. I can dance for very short periods of time. Which is hard because I used to dance for hours. So it's been really hard to lose a lot of my flexibility. I do stretch, but that's one activity that I really miss.

The alteration of my identity as that person who does everything has taken place. And being nurse, and just feeling loved by God and family, I know I don't have to be that person. So I have to talk to myself about not being proud. And, you know that it's ok. I have no patience. If there's something I can do, I will do it, a hundred percent. Physical therapy, whatever, I am an "A" student in anything.

So, after I had had so much pain in the back of my neck due to micro-fractures in my cervical vertebrae that that's when I was suicidal. That's the only time in my life. My mom was suicidal the whole time I was growing up, so I was used to taking care of her. And I was used to her saying things like, "I'm going to lock myself in the garage and turn on the car". Thank you mother. I'm 10 years old. I really want to know this. So that had always been a last option for me.

I started seeing a neurologist about 5 or 6 years ago when I was having the problems on the Viox. Because I'd been having headaches with all this. I've had migraines in the past, not too many in the last 10 years or so. But, you know, with the fluorescent lights and the computer – and I'd be on the computer and it would trigger. And I'd get the scintillating scartoma, they call it. The little flashing lights, usually on one side. And occasionally I'll get the dark holes where I can see around the perimeter but I can't see straight in front of me.

The last 3 years, my sister, a massage therapist, started working on me. And for 2 years I was getting pretty much weekly massages. And she's worked on me for like an hour and a half or two hours. And that helped a lot. And I think it had permanent benefit. It's on-going. She moved so I haven't been getting those. And I've been to a massage therapist at home and she's a good generic massage therapist and it helps but I really miss having my sister work on me, a lot. And I having to use my traction device a lot more.

I can do meditation and I have some relaxation exercises. I used to teach stress management and relaxation classes. Cognitive trial which is real good. Thought stopping followed by physical relaxation followed by imagery. And I've done that enough that I can relax pretty quickly. I use heat packs a lot. Cold for anything but an injury, I don't tolerate cold at all. I can't swim in a cold pool; I just stiffen up so badly.

It's hard for me to slow down, but I'm learning to do that. I stretch some every day. I use heat for about 15 or 20 minutes. And then I start my stretching, especially with my shoulder. And I do all my stretching lying down and I find that is the biggest help. I'm a lot better now about taking breaks.

So now I have my regimen of heat, stretching, rest. And then I'll work about 2 hours; usually around the house or whatever I'm doing and then stretch out again. I have to get horizontal frequently and take the burden, weight off my back. Gravity by itself hurts by standing. I used to do yoga and I loved that. But there's very little I can do anymore. I don't have very much flexibility. I've just kinda learned to control my life a lot better, and have to limit some of my activities.

I do imagery, I do pray for people. If it's real hard for me to focus and the pain level is high, it seems like when I start praying for other people that I can focus on that and then I start relaxing. And it's like that's a technique I've learned that works for me a lot. I also have this technique that I focus on parts of my body that don't hurt. And I focus on the places that don't hurt. And I think it comes from doing self-hypnosis. I'm trained in clinical hypnosis. I just kinda concentrate on finding something that is ok and to take the focus away from the negative and I've done that with my whole life.

I feel like I'm one of those people who have maximized and capitalized on everything I have going for me and that that's one way I've been able to stay really functional. And a sense of humor. Lord, you've got to have sense of humor. And support. And my husband now really takes good care of me. And he's very understanding. I don't complain very often unless something unusually bothering me and I am so.

A lot of my condition is so barometric pressure related and weather related. It's like that's 80% - 90%. So I'll watch the weather channel and I look for the next sunny day coming. I remember years ago I used to get up and take hot baths when I ached in the middle of the night, because pain would wake me up fairly frequently. So I'm going to take that time. And I can do that. Because I'll have couple days when I'll feel better and I know I can get something done. Sometimes I change the schedule for an appointment of something I need to do.

Lily   Age: 41

A typical day in my life is very busy. I have 2 boys, my husband works long hours. I am a part time hairdresser at home, and I started working for a greeting card company. My day is pretty hectic, pretty much on an everyday basis.

I was diagnosed with FM about 12 years ago. I was having problems with my jaw, and I thought it was from a dental appointment, and I did see an ear, nose and throat specialist that my children had been to many, many times. And, they diagnosed the TMJ with the fibromyalgia. My family doctor kind of confirmed it. I was a full time hairdresser, you just think that's because you're tired so I never questioned it. You don't feel good and you go to the doctor and there's nothing wrong. Well after a while you quit going to the doctor. So I didn't really pursue it at that point. When I had the problem with my jaw. I couldn't move it. That's when I went to the ear nose and throat specialist. Then I went to my family doctor and he kind of confirmed, and then we stared on all the different things to do.

I research everything, so I read every book there was to read about it. I did try the low dose antidepressants at night to help me sleep. I tried naproxin and you know, pain medicines like that, over the counter. I did start taking an antidepressant, it is supposed to help you quit smoking, and I was on it for a while. Even though I didn't quit smoking I didn't have any headaches. So I asked my doctor if I could stay on it because by being on that I didn't have to take aspirins or anything like that. So that worked really well until we changed insurance and then I can't take that unless I go see a shrink. So I don't take that anymore. So I do have the headaches again.

I researched guafenesin; there's a book out now about guafenesin treatment, and that worked really well for me, it's the only thing that really worked for me. It just kind of keeps you on an even keel. You still deal with the pain on a daily basis. I find that even though I hate the heat, when it's warmer out, I am better. And I don't know if it's the liquid in your body and your muscles are more fluid, do you know what I mean? But I know in the colder weather, or the rainy weather, I have a harder time with the muscle pain.

For me I guess you just deal with it, like somebody who has arthritis. They have the pain. It's maybe not constant all day long. But sometimes I just have to say no, and just quit doing, and just sit down and read a book or something, you know, to relax a little bit. And then there are certain things that I can't do. Like I can't sit in the car for any long periods of time, I get too sore just sitting there. I don't know, I just try to stay busy and not think about it much. You do have your days, and your moments, and things that you are limited to, but basically that's where I am at. I think that once you have it and have it for long enough, people get sick of your complaining and hearing about how you feel so you don't talk about it, you just deal with it.

I tried an exercise program, but it bothers me a lot. It makes me more sore, so when I do try and exercise I have to go really slow. I can't lift heavy weights and things like that, or exert, 'cause it puts me back then. I have too much pain. I do go for a massage every six weeks. That really helps.

There's different things that I do at home when I have the pain. I have a problem with my back, and I'll get these knots up in the muscles in my back, so my massage therapist recommended that I try to take a hard ball, like a tennis ball and you lay on it.

Well, I lay on it; I don't go up against the wall. I just lay on the floor, I put it there and it hurts but once you start pushing some of that fluid out of that muscle, and then you move your body on that ball so that you're kind of working it off, like say if someone is working on your back. And that works really good for me.

I use hot pads a lot. Hot baths work really well for me. I know it's hard to do that in the summer. I try to swim. I'm not a good swimmer but I try to exercise in the pool, because there is a little less resistance on the muscles. My legs are a problem. But also, you're a hairdresser, you stand all day long, you are always on your feet. So that sometimes is a problem.

I think just accept the fact that you have it and it's something that you're going to deal with it the rest of your life, that's pretty much the easier part of it. You are still going to have it; you're still going to have problems. But once you get past that I think it's just easier to deal with. Your family understands a little bit better some of the things that you get with it.

Self-knowledge is a big one. Just learning as much as you can. I did go to a class. It was through the Arthritis Foundation and it was like an 8-week course. That was very good because then you get to exchange ideas, and people that are just coming in and they don't really know a lot about it, then their telling their story, and then you are trying to help them – "no, you don't want to do this, and don't want to do that…he doesn't know what he's talking about, etc.

I think the more you learn and you're able to talk to other people that have it its easier. Because people who don't have it don't understand it, they think you're nuts. They don't know how you feel inside.

It might be attitude because I have more of a 'you can kiss my butt' attitude now. When people kind of take advantage and that kind of thing. I'm always there to do everything for everybody and sometimes that is overlooked and you're not appreciated. So I do have more of that where I blow off a little more instead of letting it bother me emotionally. And that's good. I've had a lot of stressful things in my life the last year and that I think has helped me. Because as long as I can maintain my own then I won't let other people take advantage of me so much. So that has helped a lot. I say it different in my head but 'kiss my butt' attitude is what I would call it. So, it's almost like you stand up for yourself a little bit more. And that's better for me, instead of being the doormat.

    I think they should research as much as they can, be open with their doctors because most doctors are very alert about fibromyalgia. And if you have a better communication – because a lot of the times you go to the doctor and you don't really know if you have the flu or if it's the fibromyalgia flaring up then.

    And I think probably learn what your limitations are. Learn that, because once you can learn that, then you can take care of yourself better. When you need to rest, you rest. If you need to cancel something, you cancel. Because you don't feel good. You don't just keep pushing, pushing all the time. And that's what most people do. They don't want to accept that they have a limitation maybe and so if they push themselves hard enough they think they can overcome kind of on their own, and they can't.

    Well with the fibromyalgia you have the muscle pain and the soreness and the fatigue you lot of times have, you know, irritable bowel syndrome kind of goes with that, the headaches I recently developed a skin sun sensitivity. So I don't know if its age or it has anything to do with anything. I have to watch that in the sun.

    And I think that there is just so many things that go with it that you could put it all in one category. If you don't have them all you pretty much have a lot of them. You have to be careful with things that you eat, and things that you do and all of that. That's what makes it a little more complex because each person has a lot of those. They think they have fibromyalgia and that's why they go to the doctor and if the doctor's don't recognize it then they say they don't. I saw a rheumatologist; he did not diagnose me. He didn't think I had it. Which is fine, that's what he's supposed to do. He's supposed to be the thorough one.

I was in a car accident and I didn't have my seatbelt on. I didn't get hurt badly; I just got banged up. I heard other people say that there was this traumatic thing that happed. Whether there was an accident. Or working out too much, people can get it from working out too much. They can injure those muscles and not regain it back. So, I often question that because I had my accident, say 5 years before I was diagnosed. So I don't know if it played a part in it.

Petunia   Age: 37

I get up about 8 o'clock and I spend about half an hour every day getting ready. I generally take medicine as I'm going out the door and I eat in the car on my way to work. I try to eat like a protein bar. A lot of my day is sitting and typing so it's kind of stressful. So I make sure I get up and take a break and stretch and do weird little exercises for me, I don't really care about other people. But I try to walk around and just move.

I try to keep more of a schedule and try to keep things routine so that I'm not throwing myself off and doing things that aren't messing up the schedule that I have which will contribute to pain or discomfort or any of that kind of stuff. The healthy piece of me is that I've become more aware of what I need and what does hurt me and what does feel better and try to use it to my advantage.

I think I was diagnosed with fibromyalgia when I was 25. And after that point I was basically in college. So I was walking around all the time, and dancing all the time, basically physically active. I think that's when I went into the real world and actually started sitting more and not exercising as much, I started to notice all my aches and pains and the problems that I have. So I went to doctors and some of them I think really didn't get that all the symptoms were together. And when I found somebody that did, I was kind of relieved that they put a name to it. And actually said, yeah, it's not all in your head. Even though they still at the time kind of alluded to – well if you take anti-depressants you'll just be better. And, you know, it's kind of like a neurotic physically condition, that women have or something.

And then the more I continued working and being more sedentary in later 20's it became harder. Because I was getting more and more pain. And I already had arthritis too. So I was getting to the point where I was going to doctors, and getting medications and getting physical therapy and things like that. I went through a lot of medications, that helped some but they didn't help a lot. After a while I started feeling like a guinea pig, and I was gaining a little bit of weight. Basically I think I was in denial about how bad it was getting, and I started to feel like I didn't have control over it. So I was getting very depressed and unhappy about it.

And there' some other things in my life that weren't very positive at the time. Once I got to a point where I kind of hit bottom with I'm just too negative, I'm just too depressed and there has to be some control I have over it I felt better. I finally got to a point where I just came back up and finally realized that I have control over it as long as I manage most of it. And that sometimes I will need medicine and sometimes I don't need medicine. But probably if I do all I can do, that I can minimize the amount of medication that I need and just be better. I have a more positive thought about it.

I don't really think they really know what it does to you in the long term. I worry about that. I worry about my liver and my kidneys and cancer and this buildup of junk in my system. And know you can't really get away from it, because of the way we live in general. But I do know if I can minimize what I'm contributing to it, that maybe it will help so that I don't get cancer. Maybe I can die a natural death.

I'm not a religious person, and I don't attend church and I don't really pray and that kind of stuff. I do think there's a difference between being spiritual and religious and I might consider myself a little bit spiritual but I don't have anything specific set for that per se. I try to take care of my mental health, spiritual health; I network with a lot of people professionally. Having a lot of those resources just reduces my stress, in relation to my job. Which is really my focus in life.

I try to stay around healthier people, more positive people. Internally I try to fight my negative tendency of thoughts, and things like that, by trying to read more positive things. I think knowledge is power. I think to learn more about what's wrong with you, what issue you have, you have more power to manage it or do something about it. Even if it's not going to change you can still decide how you want to think about it differently.

I guess internally I just think I'm a strong person and I have a lot of strong will, and I basically have always had the money. So if there's something I want to do I'll do it. I don't let a lot of things hold me back. I also try not to be emotionally restrictive. If I feel like crying, and I'm upset about something I just try to go with it. I don't try to be ridiculous and over dramatic, but I don't want to hold it in. I have journaled before, and if I'm really upset I'll write things down, but I don't do that on a regular basis. I try to be aware of me and my responses to things, and everybody else in general, which I think, helps to keep me healthier.

    I said things like: this can't continue, I can't live like this, I refuse to live like this forever, because if this is how I have to live the quality of life is bad, I don't like it. And I just refused to totally give into it. Because I know I have more control over things. I can't get rid of it; there's no cure for it. But I still think that I have a lot more control of the situation. Even I if can't make myself physically feel better by exercising or whatever. I can still approach it mentally from the perspective that I can still control how I want to respond to it.

    So, I think I basically got sick of myself. And I think that my husband was getting sick of me and my complaining. And I'm one of those people that complains. I have to complain. My blood pressure goes up. You know, I just have to say it and just have to say it and I have to say it the way I need to say it and in the amount of time I need to say it or else I don't feel like I've resolved it. But I got sick and tired of myself complaining and feeling that way and feeling miserable and if you don't like it this way then change it. So that's what I was trying to do.

    And I think it's one of those things that I've changed and I've evolved and it gets better and gets worse. It's kind of a cycle, but at the same time I think what I realized about it was that nobody really seems to stay the same and we're getting older. You have to constantly evolve with things. So, I guess I just have a lot of awareness of – if you decide not to do something then it's your own fault if you're not better now. You feel worse now because you're not doing what you should be doing to meet where you're at, at the time. So, that's pretty much been my self-talk and my continued self-talk is you know. You have to do your part in it if you want to feel better. And just realizing that I have a lot of control over it.

    I don't think it ever goes away. But there have been times, there have been a couple days, in my life, maybe a holiday, oh-my-god, I'm not in any pain at all, and this is weird. And then I start thinking about it, and wouldn't it be nice to know what a normal person's life is like. 'Cause I just assume that everybody feels crappy like I do every day. And I imaging that being without any pain seems like a fantasy to me. But at the same time, it has to be a reality because some people my age seem to be able to something's that I can't do. Or I have to do them in a restricted way then they do them.

    I would like to not have the problem. Not have any pain, and the arthritis and TMJ and everything else like that. I know it's unrealistic, it's never going to be there. I guess the way I would like it to be, I want to be able to make my exercise routine, and the way that I live and that I eat. Be more healthy and be more automatic so that I don't have to think about doing it every day. I just do it and know it's a part of my life. And also have it be to where I don't measure the amount of pain that I'm in day today. Oh today's a 7 on a scale of 1 to 10, that being bad. Or, today's a 3. I want to just be able live my life and know I have it under control and not really have to reflect on every single day. Medicine free if possible as well.

    When I was diagnosed, it was more of a relief to me. Despite that fact that it was negative and it was still kind of the hysterical woman kind of thing. It's all in your head. I still felt that somebody recognized that I have something that was legitimate. And after I was diagnosed. I also found a different doctor, I found a better doctor. And since I've had him as a doctor he has been very attentive to what I say. He believes me. And it's important to be believed. I think he wants to help me and listens to what I say. And I get the referrals I need from him. If I need a referral for physical therapy or occupational or whatever – it's done. Everything, chiropractic, acupuncture medicine, exercise, etc.

But also I guess when I was diagnosed I didn't feel – it wasn't a surprise to me cause I always felt like I had a dysfunctional body. Like I had a body that kind of came out damaged at the start - my head, the jaw surgery, and my jowls out of alignment. I didn't see a therapist till many years later. I've also been in a lot of like fender bender car accident kind of things where I've never had any major injuries. I've only had bruises, or when I was younger a tooth knocked out or something like that. But I think it's impacted how I felt. I think it's no surprise to me that there was something wrong. I finally just had to get somebody figure out what the something was as a whole.

I guess the other thing that was a relief to me was that it was - all the little things wrong with me were actually the one thing. That made me feel better. I'm not a hypochondriac because my neck hurts, and my knee hurts, and my elbow. You know, it's a whole system of problems that's one problem. That actually helped me to feel better too, I think. And over time I had to feel like it's the big issue in terms of do you have any conditions, or – I don't people really understand that it's a holistic thing of problems that affects you in many different ways. Whether it's gastrointestinal or mental or something else.

I heard a lot of: you don't look handicapped. You're not, and yet there are days when I feel like it. I feel like I'm handicapped. And other days I'm normal. And even the days I feel kind of handicapped I still consider myself normal, but there's a lot of different facets of this problem that I continue to learn about and have different responses for sometimes at different times.

Rose   Age: 41

I used to be a lot more active. I was into sports a lot; I played a lot of tennis. I used to do some jogging, and liked indoor exercise stuff. I belonged to a gym and stuff like that. After my son was born is when things started kinda going downhill. That was over 13 years ago. I was able to keep up more with the housework then. I didn't really have problems with getting on the floor and scrubbing the floors and vacuuming and all that kind of stuff. I have a hard time remembering what it was like to do that. I was overall a lot more active, whether with just taking care of the house, or exercising, or work. I didn't get as worn out from working all day. I had enough energy to go out in the evening.

Actually when I found out that I had fibromyalgia I was elated because somebody had finally put a name on it. 'Cause I had - what I hear is pretty common – I had gone for years to different doctors, and they would do all sorts of tests and everything would come back negative. And I would get the thing; "maybe you're just depressed", ''cause that was also probably about the time when it was just starting to kick in when somebody would say fibromyalgia, and they'd go – what? Um, 'cause it was like you know, for a lot of things I would be like borderline on test, or just – they didn't know what to call it.

So, I would just trudge around dragging and have to deal with people thinking that I was just lazy, like my husband sometimes. So I did one of those 1-

800-doctor things and came up with a rheumatologist that just happened to be familiar with fibromyalgia and had done some research on it. And when he was asking me questions all of a sudden a lot of the things that seemed totally unrelated were all lumped together under this one thing. And he was doing the trigger points and all that. I about hit the ceiling on all of them. And he said: "Well, I think you have fibromyalgia." And it was just like 'whew'! I went home and I was so happy. I was like - I do have something! 'Cause I was just getting tired of doctors and whoever thinking that it was just something in my head.

We tried some medication, which actually is probably the meds I am still on. And that made a really big difference in itself. Now there were other things that he had mentioned that I would have liked to, but I didn't try because insurance didn't want to cover it. Like deep massage therapy and whirlpool stuff, and that kind of occupational therapy stuff, and acupuncture. But I didn't do any of that, because just like I say, insurance didn't want to cover it, so.

But it did make quite a difference, just even with the meds. 'Cause before that I was just so exhausted and hurting so bad all the time and my son was little, he was only like 1 or 2. But there would be times when much to my horror, I would doze off and all of a sudden wake up and think: "Oh, my god, where's Nick?" 'Cause you know, it was just like you would be sitting up and trying so hard to stay awake and just forcing yourself, but it was you literally could not stay upright. It was just horrendous. And if I would sit on the floor with him or something. There was no way I could get up. I would have to call somebody. So I couldn't be on the floor with him. It was just awful. But I remember especially with that being tired stuff, which I am still tired, but not to the extent where I'm falling asleep when I have my baby there. That just horrified me. So, the medication did seem to help that.

And he did mention like a regular exercise thing to improve it, which I had tried on and off. But it would hurt so much to exercise that, you know I would eventually wind up just giving it up. Just 'cause - if you know something is going to hurt, you don't do it. I would try to stick it out and then... I used to walk a lot too. And sometimes, like I still had been to the gym for a short time after that, and when I would go and try to work out for a couple of hours, just like weight training and stuff, I would come home and would just lay on my bed on my back and just with tears, running out of my eyes because it hurt so bad all over. Like I say, it doesn't take a brick to fall on my head, I just can't keep this up. So I realize it's something that may have helped but I didn't stick with it. I admit it.

Just hearing the diagnosis of fibromyalgia – which in itself didn't make me change things. But having it, I just couldn't be as active as I was. Which really bothered me because I had always liked getting out and like I say, things like playing tennis and all that. And I couldn't play with my son when he was really little. I mean I would play with him but I didn't have the energy as much as I wanted to play with him and that in itself was kinda depressing. Instead of them saying my depression was causing it, it was causing depression. I mean not to the point where I crawled into a hole, but it just bothered me that I couldn't do as much as I wanted to do.

I try to sleep better. Because if I don't get enough sleep it just makes everything worse. And actually, the last little over 4 months I have been on C-pap myself because I had really severe sleep apnea. And since I've been on that it's also helped me sleep better which in turn helps the fibromyalgia somewhat. I do try to eat better, a little. It's not always the case. I just kinda do what I've gotta do.

Well, one thing, going back with the lifestyle

change. One thing that – I mean there were many reasons that I switched and went back to school and wanted to do the sleep studies. But one of the many reasons was that I used be in special Ed and I was a teacher's aide. And it was really physical work 'cause I was with the severely delayed kids. Delayed, like mentally disabled. But also physically disabled and medically fragile. Our class was like from 8 year olds up to like 14. And so they could get pretty big. And they were in wheel chairs and we would have to change them and always be doing 2 person lifts for positioning and lifting. And I noticed, it just was wearing on me too much. Every year that we would go back to school it was like I would notice that I was slowing down a little bit more and things started acting up more, so far as muscle soreness and my back going out and that kind of stuff. So one of the reasons that I switched careers overall was because it was just too physically demanding.

   One way of taking care of myself was switching jobs. I don't how much I would say inner healing. I do try to have some time to myself and sometimes I like to just be quiet and think. Not in a formal sense of meditation, but just kind of be outside on my own. One thing that I really, really like is that part of my drive to work is going through the forest preserves, past Maple Lake and all that. And I just love going through there, and especially when I come home in the morning, when it's real early and the mist will be on the lake, and you're driving through the tress. And sometimes you'll see a deer – although I saw a dead deer this morning. The live ones are nicer! But as you drive through there you think: "I am glad I am alive to see this." There was one time I came home, in March or whenever it was when we had that freaky snow and the trees hadn't had all their leaves on or anything and just all the snow on it. It was just gorgeous. So when I drive through there it's just like: "Thank you, God, that was so nice." Yeah, things like that kind of keeps me going. Things that just make me smile inside.

    If I were free of the health problem I would clean the house from top to bottom. Which I am trying in bits and pieces but I just wear out. Yard work, I would do. Now it's like where I'll trim 2 bushes and I collapse and it just makes me really mad. Because I know it needs to be done, I want it to be done; I don't like it when it's not done. And I would probably redo the yard. Organize the house from top to bottom. Clean it. I would be out playing tennis.

    I would like to able to go out and hang out with my son some more. He likes to play ball and stuff like that with us. I try to but it's just really exhausting. I would probably cook more dinners. I would probably work some overtime. There's something that at work, they were just mentioning about starting a support group for like people with C-pap and that. They're looking for somebody do run and organize that. And that's something that I would like to do but I know there's no way I would have it in me to do it. So that's something else that I would like to do. I think a major improvement is just making a career switch. Because now I am in something that uses more of my head and is not so much physically demanding.

    Trying to get the better sleep. Sticking with my medications. Like I said, it kind of like I do what I've gotta do. I don't know how successfully I am with it but I am definitely better then when I started it probably a lot of pieces of things that have headed that way. But I think primarily, initially anyway, the medication was what got me out of that initial rut where I just couldn't stay awake. I just wouldn't be able to get out of bed at that time. I could actually sleep for; I could sleep probably for an entire weekend and still be sore and icky. That is just kind of like you just get tired of hurting all the time. It would just be nice to be able to do something and know that I could do a second thing without having to blow my next 2 days. Like I was saying, if I go out and I do some yard work or something, I might as well write off the next couple of days because I'll be too sore and exhausted to go on until I recharge for a while. Like a really slow recharge.

I just try and do whatever I can and I've tried to change my attitude to quote; "Not sweat the small stuff". And if the house is a mess, it bothers me yes, but I just do what I can and I figure that's all that I can do. I just try to not fret over things that don't matter in the big picture. Which has helped somewhat. Because if I am allowing myself to say its ok, that I don't do this or this. Then I don't feel like I'm missing that much. So it's like a shift in attitude too.

I would say if you know that you feel like you have something wrong, that something isn't right, don't let doctors write you off. And you may just be spinning your wheels if you're trying to get the same doctor to change his mind. 'Cause they're not going to do it. Ask people for recommendations if they know and doctors that are familiar with it. And just keep trying different doctors until you find someone who knows what they're doing. Because it is something totally real and it came be improved but it's your job to go out and track down somebody who can help. And I am glad I wound up – mine was sorta just dumb luck – that I came up with a doctor who knew what he was doing. But I am really glad I did because at least then you have an ally and somebody you can go to and can refine your treatment, and get it to where you can actually live a little instead of look at your bedroom ceiling all day. That's my story and I'm sticking to it.

Violet   Age: 65

I've had signs of this since I've been in my twenties. I'll just have to say, in my youth, in my teenage years, in my earlier 20's and 30's. I was very active. I was married at 20. I had 2 kids. I bowled twice a week. They were just a year apart, so it was quite active. Friendly with the neighbors, and we did a lot of work on our home and I helped my husband with that a lot. I even tried golfing, and when I look back now I can tell why I could barely make it through the 6th hole was because of this.

But I did have arthritis, so I was blamed for arthritis. My mother had rheumatoid arthritis, so I assumed it was that. Nothing tending towards, you know. But even when I went back to work I was pretty active. I could kinda run through the halls at work and when I saw someone, I would slow down. And then it just became increasingly worse. But I'm an active person in my mind, it's just my body is not going along with it.

Well, I really thought I had it even when I had arthritis. I brought an article to the doctor and I said gee, could I have this 'cause I have all the symptoms. He said, well yes, you could have it, you know, because of what I had described to him. I had been going to him for a while. But he said you're not the personality for it. Evidently, they think people should be depressed or maybe they're depressed then. And they feel like they have something wrong or maybe they had something wrong and they become depressed. I'm not sure what their attitude is toward it.

I had talked to two other people that said why don't you try these doctors downtown which I did. And then I was officially diagnosed with it. But I was getting so tired at work that when no one was around I would put my head down, and when somebody was around I would try to act alert. So, it wasn't too shocking. They tried all these antidepressants which are supposedly a painkiller, slight painkiller. And you take it just before you go to bed, and also to help you sleep. I never was very good at staying asleep, or even getting asleep. And it could be from this but it was just the way I was as long as I can remember. So, none of those worked. I tried all of them. You try them for a few months. It was just the going back and forth to the doctor. To me it was a waste of time. It might help someone else but it did absolutely nothing for me. I was even later on put on naproxin. Absolutely nothing, did nothing for me. I tried ibuprofen, which supposedly doesn't help it.

    I went to a doctor because of pain in my hip thinking maybe it was the bone and he said let's try prednisone. Well, my heart was pounding, I thought I was having a heart attack one time. So when I went back to rheumatologist, he said it does nothing for it, which of course, it didn't. The only time I got any help was about maybe 7 years ago. The sciatic nerve on my left leg got so severe that I could not stand it. I could not sleep it was so severe. So I went back to the rheumatologist, who was downtown. And I don't drive downtown. So anyhow, I went back to him. "Is there anything new that you can give me". Nothing, nothing helps and this is unbearable pain. I'm used to living with pain, so I just forge ahead." So he put me on ultram, and that's the only thing that has helped. I'll take it - I've tried to cut down on it. I take it twice a day, two pills twice a day. And try to cut down in the evening, because I do take medication to help me sleep.

    It just became so hard and I was working, I had a hard time getting up and getting ready. And then trying to pretend I was doing all right. Words were escaping me, because I was so tired, and to concentrate. I finally had to decide I have to quit work. I just absolutely couldn't do it anymore. So it did. I kinda watch my grandchildren because we live right by them, right next door. So when they came home from school we were there for them. You know, you feel that you're being productive. This was 13 years ago.

And I still try to push myself to do things but I'm so limited. I have to stay asleep in the morning, if I wake up I have to stay in bed, wait for the pills to work. It's not that I take... like I say, the second set of pills. When I start feeling better. It's only if something that's absolutely scheduled can I really force myself. And of course, once you're forcing yourself you can do it. But you cannot do this every day, all day long.

So I did go back this last year and a half, maybe two now, to bowling just once. But I am having a harder time because the arthritis is acting up and I'm just exhausted when it's over. Whenever I do something, no matter how small it is, 'cause it takes me a while to do anything... if I do anything, even get ready to go out. May be just sit, go out to a movie, or go out – I play silly cards or bunco – then I'm beat the next day, more so than usual. The exhaustion absolutely never goes away.

I do have chronic fatigue. I'm tired from chronic fatigue. The pills do not affect me at all. And any pills that possibly would affect me I take right before I go to sleep, so I wouldn't know if it's doing that. How do I cope? I just cope because it's not in my nature to give in to anything. So I just make myself do things. But, I know that I'm limited, that why I don't wear myself out with insignificant things. You know, like cleaning the house every day or doing something like that. So I limit myself, and I save my energy for what I'm going to do. I'll try to lay around a little bit more when I know I'm going out to golf that evening. I just time it around... because I'm 65 now I think I deserve to have social life. Where very easily you could just lay in bed.

I do, like on Sundays, when my husband is working across the street, and so are my kids. So, I just lay in bed, watch the movies and read the paper, and do things like that. Even though that's tiring also. You know, anything you do is tiring, just using your eyes. I'd say I just cope because that's my mindset. If I were free of it I don't know if I'd still be working right now. But I would continue to work. A lot of my friends also go out a little more often and play bridge and I learned how to do that. I would definitely try golfing. And, I'd be a little bit more active. We have 3-year-old granddaughter here and through the years I'm just more and more tired, I would just have a little more fun playing with her. Like I did with the other one. I would just live life a little fuller, go for walks and that. But that drains my energy even though I'm supposed to be doing the walking.

I just don't... I don't enjoy life the way I should enjoy it. I should be out pushing the kids on the swing. Just doing a little bit more. I don't go shopping; my husband does all that. And once in a while, I'll go to a store, but I don't unless I'm up and ready for something else at that time. I'm not going to waste the energy to get myself ready, curl my hair, take a shower, all that, just to go out to a store. So I really don't do that. Most of my clothes are bought as gifts from my husband and the kids. When I have the energy I return them and get something else. But I have to take someone with me so I have to know my limitations in order to enjoy what I want to do.

I'd just like to say that is that it never ever goes away. People don't realize, you know, oh you look fine. Well, make-up does a lot. You don't want to go around crying about it. And of course they tease me. It would just be so nice if everyone would understand. Because you don't have something on the outside. This supposedly is a disease, or whatever, that will not kill you. You know, but it just goes on and on and on.

And I can understand why people do get depressed. I rarely get depressed, because I just won't let myself thing about it. But if I ever lay there and really think about it, I just want to cry. Because no one knows, you can't feel that my arms, everything from my head to my toes hurts. I still have the muscle strength. Except my hands, the arthritis is starting to bother me. I don't know if I have spiritual strength. It may be. It's just the way that I am. My mother had arthritis, she lived with it. She had 7 kids.

I do remember saying at one time that I did get worse after I broke my arm. I could force myself before that. But then after, I was off work and I went back to work. And my husband said, why don't you just work. I said let's wait through the summer and see how it was. So that could have exacerbated it. So I think that might have added to it, like now I have to stop doing this stuff. I just can't push it, where I could live with it much more before. But I was working for about 15 years. So you go to work, and you're sitting at your desk, I did do the running around. But after a while I was like dragging around. So I would say it makes it ah… the trauma added to it.

You know how sometimes it's an effort to breathe. Here all along, this isn't all the time. But at different times, it's not just the chest hurting on top, it's just this weakness when you breathe. It just such an effort, just to breathe.

And when I feel like that, then I feel sick. Your head is woozy; your whole body feels almost like it's sick. That's the only way I can describe it. You know, it's not just the muscles and all that, it's all inside of you. But when it's an effort to breathe, like you can't force yourself to do anything. And I think that's how maybe some people who are more insecure feel more often.

"Who are you?" said the caterpillar...
"I hardly know, sir, just at present", Alice replied rather shyly.
"At least I know who I was when I got up this morning,
But I think I must have been changed several times since then."
  - Lewis Carroll, Alice in Wonderland

Chapter 8. Journeying on the Wellness Path

Being diagnosed with an illness can quite understandably produce massive confusion. Like waking up in a strange country to which one does not remember traveling, and may well feel that they do not know what to do or whom to turn for help, according to Myss (1997). A closed mind is not an asset. Be open to any and every option that can help. It has become popular in alternative healing circles to take a negative view of allopathic medicine. Strong negative feelings about or fears of allopathic medicine are not a good reason to rule them out. One's healing efforts can end up as attempts to run away from conventional medicine more than as attempts to run toward the improvement of one's health. Keep in mind that in many cases; the most effective course of action is to combine the best of both worlds.

Whole health is, in part, the result of a harmonious flow of energy between our physical and mental selves. When this flow is thrown out of balance for any reason, the body and mind react to one another rather than act cooperatively. Negative emotions, beliefs and attitudes such as lack of self-love, powerlessness, resentment, and anger can overwhelm the cerebral self, causing traumatic energy to be directed into the body. It responds by taking steps to organically expel the energy that has burdened it, and expressing it by means of physical symptoms such as illness, fatigue, or disease.

In some cases, these symptoms can simply be allowed to run their natural course and recovery will come about naturally. Usually health and wellness can only be restored by a combined course of treatment that acknowledges both the physical signs of energy clearing and the underlying emotional causes.

Self-management has increasingly been recommended as part of standard care for fibromyalgia, according to Rooks et al. (2007). Walking, simple strength training movements, and stretching activities improve functional status, key symptoms, and self-efficacy in women with fibromyalgia actively being treated with medication. The benefits are enhanced when combined with targeted self-management education. The findings suggest that appropriate exercise and patient education be included in the treatment of fibromyalgia. I would add to the treatment of all chronic pain conditions.

It's so important to be in your body, to understand the workings of your mind, to listen to and trust your feelings, and to be as conscious as you can be in your relationships, your work, in everything you do. You have to become committed to your healing journey. When a need for a more balanced life becomes very strong within you, you'll be less interested in giving energy to the beliefs and expectations, the fears and judgments that supported it and helped maintain its hold over you. Your fear of not really living will become stronger that the fear of stepping out, of risk taking. (Dreaver, 1996).

According to Braden (2011) electrical and magnetic energy form the atoms of matter. A change in the energy changes the atoms. Our hearts produce the strongest electrical and magnetic energy of the body. Heart-based feelings or beliefs create electrical and magnetic waves that extend into the world beyond our bodies. As we change our beliefs, we change the energy that forms the atoms of our world.

All of us experience varying degrees of problems in our lives. Illness, whether of the physical body or the mind and emotions, is one type of negative experience. Every challenge or problem you face is negative energy, according to Grayson (1997). But no problem is insurmountable, no illness incurable. Negative experiences exist, but they have no fundamental reality. They are inversions of truth or primal nature. All negative experiences can be neutralized, and to think otherwise is thinking from a limited point of view.

The medical profession admits that there is always more to learn and to discover. No one knows all and this is the fountain of hope for everyone. Illness, malfunctions and disorders are inverted action caused by a distorted or disturbed consciousness and manifest as a disordered experience. Every problem is a temporary state of consciousness that expresses a mind/emotion pattern operating through the physical life of the individual. You're not consciously aware of the action. You always have a choice, whether to give in to negative emotions about the problem or crises or to deal with it and then let it go.

Disorders and negative experiences occur, but the average person lives life on the surface continually manipulated by these consciousness factors that are rarely neutralized because they do not understand what is happening or how to take charge of their lives. This can be changed through spiritual knowing in directed spiritual treatment. Most disorders and problems arise from unconscious factors. They are the result of some hurt, shock or trauma in personal experience, or these in combination with influences from their collective consciousness. They do not understand how to take charge of their lives and they cannot comprehend why things happen to them. We can learn that there is a consciousness factor within us and we can learn we can be in control.

    Brain receptive tissues are present throughout the body. Healing begins when we discard our ideas that we are limited creatures and realize our unbounded nature of self. We condition ourselves to believe in our own boundaries. All approaches to healing create an opportunity for healing. Illness creates a situation that demands we evaluate how we are taking care of ourselves, where we are going in life, and what is most important to us. We can support the process of reestablishing a healing balance that may enhance our innate healing powers.

    One of the profound discoveries that I made while doing the research was the discussion on *accountability.* Jahnke (1999) believes that being accountable for honesty, purposeful work, joyfulness, service, family time, and play is one of the most potent tools for improvement of health or personal performance, because it means one will do what they say they will do. It is identical to integrity.

    Accountability in self-healing practice is actually doing the practice. Jahnke says that so many times one hears that a disease has been a gift to someone, or it is the most important thing that has ever happened to me. Why would they say that? An explanation is: when people reach the point where they are no longer willing to be victims, when they become accountable for the quality of their experience, they are reborn, transformed. At that point it does not matter so much if they have a particular job, whether their life is brief or lengthy. The quality of their life is radically improved; guilt, worry, and uncontrollable fear have been cast out. Joy and trust can be purposefully invited to enter their lives. It does not matter so much what is happening. How they react to what is happening becomes the focus, and the richness of their life expands.

Accountable for the nature of their experience, they can elect to banish frustration, fear, and the torment of continuous stress. They enter a new life where they literally radiate, and enthusiasm can flourish. Those who master accountability are reborn through their own labor. Biologically this rebirth produces a fantastic medicine within the human system. Together with the health enhancement and self-healing methods, accountability is an astounding force. Accountability in relation to the self-healing methods produces vigilant practice, and vigilant practice make miracles possible (Jahnke, 1999).

I surmise that accountability is one of the things that took place within each of the women in this study. The study suggests a need for improved provider communication strategies and screening measures assessing distress and symptoms. Future research should evaluate creative interventions including group support and complementary therapy approaches to enhance perceived support, control and hope in this population.

According to Lipton (2005) one becomes disempowered by messages they receive. Human's subconscious minds are preprogrammed in the first 6 years of life. The subconscious is the primary mechanism that controls human life, and it plays "mental tapes." These programs must be changed, 70% of which are negative and redundant. In addition Lipton states that the nocebo's or negative messages, especially from authority figures, have a tremendous impact on an individual, which are affecting one on a cellular level (Lipton, 2005).

Most of the women in the study were told that they would never get better, or that there was not much that they could do about their condition. They were prescribed some medication and/or given one or two therapy options and dismissed, probably from the lack of knowledge or understanding on the part of the physician. Since the onset of fibromyalgia in most of these women, the medical field has made some progress in diagnosing and treating fibromyalgia patients, but the progress has been slow and limited. A profoundly hopeful synthesis of the latest and best research in cell biology and quantum physics shows that human's bodies can be changed as they retrain their thinking. Following is a synopsis of the research of Lipton (2005).

A human being's well-developed nervous systems headed by their big brain means that their awareness is more complicated then single cells. When the uniquely human minds get involved they can choose to perceive the environment in different ways, unlike single cells whose awareness is more reflexive. They can change the character of their lives by changing their beliefs. The belief that humans are frail biochemical machines controlled by genes is giving way to an understanding that they are powerful creators of their lives and the world in which they live.

Course of disease appears related to integrity of psychological defenses; patients with emotional decompensation are more likely to have rapidly progressing disease, to be more incapacitated, and to respond more poorly to medical treatment. Would further study of psychotherapeutic intervention have some role in the treatment of immunologically mediated diseases? I expect that the results of the study, with the narratives of women who have realized some success over their chronic conditions, will not only prove the success of the power of self-healing but will also give hope to many others still searching for a solution.

"A number of clinical trials are currently testing nonpharmaceutical approaches," according to Zautra (2008). "Characterization of fibromyalgia as a condition that benefits those facing chronic pain will provide a better and more hopeful future for these patients and the medical community responsible for their care" (pp. 1-2). Using the suggestions from Brody (2000) an individual can begin by practicing the following: give themselves full credit for whatever they are taking charge of, and see himself or herself as a person who takes charge and less as a person to whom unhealthy things just happen. This attitude will stoke up their inner pharmacy, build up their inner momentum and give them more motivation and will power to tackle what still remains to be done.

One of the ways to do this is by asking one's self to what extent is this disease running my life and how much am I running my life? Then assign a percentage. Think back over any small success over disease or discomfort in the past, and what things worked best at different times. Knowing this can produce a plan to build up one's mastery percentage. Set aside time each week to review the events of the past seven days and write down a new percentage score. Every few months look over those scores and see what headway is being made. (pp. 65-66).

A placebo can be any one of the suggestions included in this book, as well as using a compliment or an inspiration – anything that puts an individual in a happier state of mind and opens the thoughts of possibilities. The positive thought that one can take charge of their health and their attitude is just as important as what they actually do. By adjusting the message within themselves and outwardly taking some practical steps, they can effect a placebo response within themselves and begin to gain mastery over their condition.

    The theories and techniques of intrapersonal communication, focusing, neurolinguistic programming, psychoneuroimmunology and placebo response explored in this book are just a few chosen from the emerging fields of mind-body healing. They were chosen because of their success and provide some options for patients suffering with chronic painful conditions. Hopefully reader will seek more information into some of these for him/herself as possible healing approaches. Some of the women in this study used a form of at least one of these techniques without realizing it or giving it that particular name.

    The information in this book evidences that humans control their health, or the course of their disease without really knowing that they do. Now may be the time to learn how to recognize and use this control over illness. One should be able to use some sort of placebo instead of a pill. Conceiving of the mind and body as one means that wherever an individual puts their mind, they may be able to put their bodies. The mind may have to be fooled to reach a healthy place. Once one learns how to put it there consciously, the evidence suggests that the body may well follow.

    Research indicates that our cells are affected by negative thoughts and emotions that produce harmful chemicals. It also demonstrates the effect of positive attitude changes, mindfulness, and accountability to elicit healing chemicals to our cells. Not only can humans prevent illness, but can often improve or even heal an existing condition.

    Finally, I located a study by Dingley and Roux (2003) that epitomizes the women who participated in this. It was about the phenomenon of inner strength in women with various chronic illnesses. It demonstrated commonalties in the experiences that bridge the boundaries created by disease categorizing or individual circumstance. Their particular study explored older Hispanic women living with chronic illness. However, I believe that the interesting result of their study is also definitive of the participants in my research study.

The data analysis in the Dingley and Roux study suggested the following interrelated dimensions: "drawing strength from the past; focusing on possibilities; being supported by others, knowing one's purpose, and nurturing the spirit" (p. 21). The study contributes to a cumulative program of research on the phenomenon of inner strength, furthering theory generation, cultural awareness, and future intervention studies.

This book looked at the questions: Why do some people get sick or develop chronic conditions? Why do some people choose the try to get better? Why do people get better in spite of the seriousness of their condition, or a negative prognosis? The study endeavoured to answer the research question: What is the experience of women living with fibromyalgia who have been improving their health? Although there is no known cause or cure for fibromyalgia there are theories regarding what may lead up to it, and methods or options patients can use to improve their condition. But looking at a comparable concept, what may be the causes and the cures for fibromyalgia and other chronic conditions?

This book shows that people get sick because negative emotions such as fear, anger, anxiety, and negative stressors, cause glands such as the pituitary, endocrine, and adrenal glands to produce harmful chemicals such as dopamine, adrenaline, and cortisol that enter and weaken the cells. The interrelationship between our experiences, feelings, and body chemistry are intricate. Specific mental states effect specific glandular secretions, circulatory patterns, and organ functions. Therefore, there is probably no limit to the influencing of function and behavior by feelings and attitudes.

Accountability, self-efficacy, changing attitudes, and belief systems also play a part in turning around chronic conditions and illness. Often, one must fool their mind in order to enlist their own powers of self-healing. Using placebos, hypnosis, autosuggestion, faith healing, visualization, and positive thinking, one can begin to control their health. It does not matter what is happening, but how one reacts to what is happening that becomes the focus. Accountable for the nature of one's experience, one can elect to banish frustration, fear, hostility, sadness and the torment of continuous stress.

If one agrees to make choices that equate with joy, satisfaction, and trust, then a positive physiological response occurs throughout the body, particularly in the immune system. Health improves because positive emotions and exercises, such as laughter prayer and meditation, result in the production of calming and healing chemicals such as melatonin and seratonin, to name a few.

There is also a necessity to set a goal, to be detailed, realistic, and to set criteria for success. While this study is limited to a small number of women, their experiences illustrate the rich, diverse ways that the participants live with and attempt to conquer the multi-dimensional enigma that is fibromyalgia on a daily basis.

One would believe that pain would be socially understood and somewhat sympathized with. People cannot relate with the chronically ill since the individual is not screaming, crying or grimacing. Individuals with chronic illnesses often walk, talk and function somewhat normally so it is assumed that the pain is overstated. There is a constant struggle to try to have people know what they are going through, without seeming to search for sympathy and pity.

Living with an invisible chronic illness can mean constantly trying to redefine their condition.

They cannot keep up with the rest of the world, and yet the world sees no excuse for their lack of participation. It is often not only the disease itself that is painful, but also the emotional effects of having the illness discounted, having one's respectability and judgement questioned, and dealing with the criticisms of others. Thus, it is extremely necessary for the person with chronic illness to feel that his/her disease is validated (p. 7).

A study by Munce and Stewart (2007) provides evidence "from a large population sample that women suffer from both depression and chronic pain conditions at approximately twice the prevalence of men. Increased pain severity may play a particularly significant role for women, leading to further distress and further pain" (pp. 394-399).

Juhan (1987) asks if feeling states, attitudes, behavioral and physiological habits can start large circles of inter-related processes turning in vicious directions, might not different states, attitudes, and habits start them turning in healthy ones? And have we not somehow learned the attitudes and habits that are crippling us? And can we not learn new ones? I believe that self-efficacy plays a major role in initiating behavior change to affect health changes.

Bandura (1997) describes self-efficacy as the belief that one is capable of performing in a certain manner to attain certain goals. It is a belief that one has the capabilities to execute the courses of actions required to manage prospective situations.

Self-efficacy facilitates the forming of behavioral intentions, the development of action plans, and the initiation of action. Self-efficacy can assist relapse prevention. Self-efficacy can support the translation of intentions into action. For example, a person with high self-efficacy may engage in a more health-related activity when an illness occurs, whereas a person with low self-efficacy would harbor feelings of hopelessness. One's sense of self-efficacy can play a major role in how one approaches goals, tasks, and challenges.

Furthermore, a study by Stelter (2000) shows that body experience can be seen as the basis for the formation of the self-concept. But body experience is a 'data source' which is difficult to handle scientifically. Body experiences are based on "internal physical sensations" and are not in opposition to phenomenology, and self-concept is difficult to handle scientifically. Stelter presents an experiential approach that gives access to a new dimension of self-efficacy. "It is the feeling of 'I can' which is bodily anchored and not just a cognitive dimension. The felt meaning represents the fundamental intentionality in relation to the situation and is a fundamental expression of the person's relation to the situation" (p. 63).

I believe that this may be the explanation of why some people with chronic conditions, such as fibromyalgia seem to give in to hopelessness and despair. While others, such as the women in this study develop the motivation to try various means to cultivate a healthier lifestyle. I am of the opinion that a possible response to the research question: What is the experience of women living with fibromyalgia who have been *improving their health* is accountability and self-efficacy.

Accountability for their experience and the self-efficacy that allows them to want to improve their condition and set goals to accomplish that improvement. In restating Juhan's, Jahnke's and Bandura's views the following conclusions can be surmised.

Learning to be sick involves one's own physiological and emotional responses to certain stimuli one does not like, responses which either reinforce or add their own flavor to the potential negative consequences of noxious experiences. By the time the discomfort we are suffering becomes greater than the discomfort of changing our ways, the physical damage has already been done. It is this extreme psychological ambiguity of discomfort and pain themselves that diverts us from the real causes of or limitations and from the practical steps we could be taking to move beyond them (Juhan, 1987).

Bandura's work has determined that self-efficacy is influenced by four main factors: information and persuasion, observation of others, successful performance of the behavior, and physiological feedback. Patients seek out information and health professionals give credible sources of information and persuasion or encouragement to begin health changes. Observing others make healthy life style changes, and their own successful physical changes guide their actions.

I believe that attitude, intent, belief, and a strong spiritual connection are interrelated in the process of healing. This interaction leads to a quicker, more effective, and stable recovery.

"Our attitudes about pain contribute as much life-disrupting power as the actual painful sensations themselves. The discouraging cycle of hope, frustration, and continued pain can be as damaging to an everyday life as the pain itself."
- Ruth Buczynski, NICABM

Chapter 9. Further Exploration

This study has social meaning and implications because of the need to recognize individual narratives as part of the comprehensive approach to treatment. Methods used to treat fibromyalgia patients that are explored as a result of this research might improve the quality of life and/or health for the participants and possibly for many others dealing with a chronic condition. Many chronic illnesses are invisible; causing feelings and frustration that are different then what a person with a visible condition may experience, according to Copen (2002).

Pain acceptance is emerging as a promising complement to control-based pain management strategies and a likely approach to maintaining quality of life for chronic pain patients, according to the findings of Kratz, Davis, and Zautra (2007). They suggest that "pain patients with greater capacity to accept pain may be emotionally resilient in managing their condition. The concept of acceptance of chronic pain could potentially be expanded, modified, and applied to other limitations and adversity experienced by chronic pain patients" (pp. 291-301.

Pelletier (2002) states that "qualitative research is concerned with the subjective world. It offers insight into social, emotional, and experimental phenomena in healthcare to determine what, how, and why. Therefore, findings from qualitative research may contribute to systematic reviews, and reviewers need to consider how to incorporate them" (p. 7).

Findings have the potential to enhance the quality and salience of systematic reviews, and can help to define an intervention more precisely and contribute to the choice of outcome measure. Patients, practitioners, and procedures are complex, interactive, dynamic systems with other even larger and more complex ethical, philosophical, economic, and spiritual dimensions (Pelletier, 2002).

The study also shows the importance of understanding each fibromyalgia patient as an individual and the need for creative methods to alleviate their symptoms. It also establishes the benefit of using a qualitative applied research method for determining quality of life of fibromyalgia patients. It has social meaning and implications in particular for women who are diagnosed with fibromyalgia.

On a personal level, there is important information for the individual patient's family and friends. For the community as a whole, this information will benefit other women with the same diagnosis. This also extends to those in the medical communities who care for them. From the information gathered, could some techniques be developed from the commonality of all of the participants in this study that would benefit many? In my conversations with several medical doctors and practitioners, the same thread of concern arises.

Many professionals are now convinced that integrative therapies work and that body/mind connectiveness is the basis for many healing techniques. Often, they are able to convince their patients. However, the hardest and sometimes impossible task is to get the patient to start. Could the results of this study then be used as a tool for those practitioners?

Integrative Medicine is becoming a widely accepted option for thousands of people. Many therapies are beginning to be recognized within mainstream medicine. Integrative/Complementary health sessions are being prescribed by an increasing number of doctors, and several insurance companies are including coverage within their policies. Medicare has recently extended coverage for limited preventative treatments. Many of these women integrated complementary modalities into their responses to fibromyalgia.

There were several limitations to this study. The first of course, was the difficulty in recruiting participants as explained previously. I would have preferred a few more than the intended 15, rather than two less. Although I believe that the research reached a saturation point, it would have enriched the study to have a few more narratives and heard about a few more creative therapies used by women who decided to take control of their health.

The qualitative study had the goal of eliciting information regarding self-talk. I formulated the opinion that many fibromyalgia patients are cautious about discussing their condition, possibly due to experiences of negative input from doctors and friends and family. Several of the women said that they felt guilty for being sick and not able to take care of day-to-day expectations. Therefore, the reluctance to participate in a study within which they would describe their fibromyalgia experiences.

This study was conducted with women who were in an improved state of health and earnest about relating their experiences. This is not necessarily true of all fibromyalgia patients. Another limitation was the four open-ended non-leading questions that were asked. Although this provided me with an accurate narrative from each participant, I would like to return and ask many other questions. As this study was hermeneutic, qualitative and phenomenological in nature, it was necessary to conduct it in this manner. However, a further heuristic research study would prove to be of interest and value as well.

In a Heuristic study (Moustakas, 1994) the researcher engages in a self-inquiry and dialogue with others aimed at finding the underlying meanings of important human experiences. The deepest currents of meaning and knowledge take place within the individual through one's senses, perceptions, beliefs, and judgments. This requires a passionate, disciplined commitment to remain with a question intensely and continuously until it is illuminated or answered. The information gathered from this research, and resulting data will provide meaningful basis for further research in this area of intrapersonal communication and fibromyalgia, and also of intrapersonal communication and other chronic conditions.

This study shows there are some commonalties in this group of successful fibromyalgia "copers". Fibromyalgia syndrome evokes uneasiness in health care staff and greater attention needs to be paid to the links between the explanatory models of patients and staff, and to the interrelationship between the complex physical, psychological, and social needs of the patient. Taking a less medical but more holistic approach when drawing up new diagnostic criteria for FM might be a better match for individuals and may result in more effective treatment (Lempp, Hatch, Carville, & Choy, 2009).

Scascighini, Toma, Dober-Spielmann and Sprott (2008) believe that a standard of multidisciplinary programs should be internationally established to guarantee generally good outcomes in the treatment of chronic pain. "Future studies should more specifically focus on differential effects of treatment components and patient variables, allowing the identification of subgroups, which most probably would profit from multidisciplinary pain programs" (pp. 670-678).

Turk, Swanson, and Tunks (2008) explain that chronic pain is a prevalent and costly problem that eludes adequate treatment. Persistence affects all domains of people's lives, and in the absence of cure, success will greatly depend on adaptation to symptoms and self-management. As none of the most commonly prescribed treatment regimens are sufficient to eliminate pain, a more realistic approach will likely combine pharmacological, physical, and psychological components tailored to each patient's needs.

Limer, Nicholl, Thomson and McBeth (2007) interpret the findings from existing studies and in designing future studies of chronic pain. They state that evidence indicates that there is a genetic component to chronic widespread pain syndromes and pain sensitivity. No definitive pain susceptibility genes have yet been identified but the field is in its relative infancy compared with many complex diseases. Future gene association (GA) studies of chronic pain disorders should have adequate sample size for sufficient power to detect associations.

Appropriate information on pain status and potential environmental psychological cofounders is also required. This type of study is essential if the genetic component to chronic widespread pain etiology is to be fully elucidated (pp. 572-577).

In addition, the study provides an important tool for myself and other healthcare professionals to use in providing care for fibromyalgia patients. However, there is a need for further research into what is important to the patient in healing and coping with a chronic condition, not necessarily fibromyalgia.

I believe that a large portion of this study can be applied to any individual coping with a chronic condition. This study should be repeated ā FM☐ in a different geographic setting ā heuristic methodology. As stated above, a heuristic study would provide further insight into the lived experience of fibromyalgia with a group of participants.

Similar studies should be done with other chronic, non-lethal conditions. A quantitative study using the metathemes embedded in a questionnaire to test for commonalties and both successful and unsuccessful copers would be examined. "An increasing number of studies, including randomized clinical trials, point to safe and relatively inexpensive interventions that can improve health outcomes and reduce the need for more expensive medical treatments" (Sobel, 2000, pp. 395-396).

There is much to explore in the area of self-talk. Do people naturally improve over time just because they learn to cope better? Or do they improve better over time because they are being treated? Measuring quality of life with a quality of life questionnaire or with wait-list control are suggestions for future research. This book has shown options, but as a result of the outcome of the research, there are things that should be done. Is there an improvement in the quality of life that can be objectively measured? People say they feel better, but can you measure that either quantitatively or qualitatively and how would it be done?

A side issue for further study would be to investigate how to communicate information about actual changes in patient's self-evaluations to health care professionals and family members, because this information could be relevant to their involvement in patient's health care decisions. Although the women in the study have found ways to help themselves, the same methods do not work on everyone. Each individual needs to form his or her own plan.

In my practice, I have listened to women who have successfully tried trigger point therapy, becoming a vegan, exercise, acupuncture, and massage therapy, to name a few. However, each individual had to formulate their own combinations to realize results. It is a frustrating and often prolonged venture. Can proven methods be looked at in a systematic controlled setting?

Some Treatment Considerations for Chronic Pain
Reported by Patients
(in order of the most helpful)

Most Helpful
+ Pacing of activities
+ Avoiding chemicals
+ Massage/body work
+ Avoiding problem foods
+ Yoga, tai chi, qigong
+ CBT – cognitive behavioral Therapy
+ Change in outlook
+ Treatment for sleep
+ Narcotics for pain
+ Herbal medicines

Very Helpful
+ Other hormones
+ Graded exercise
+ Water/salt increase
+ Acupuncture
+ NADH
+ Thyroid supplements
+ Aggressive rest
+ Antidepressants
+ B-12 injections

Helpful
+ Glutathione
+ Magnet therapy
+ Teeth filling/removal
+ Beta blockers
+ Kutapressin

References

Ader, R. (1981). *Psychoneuroimmunology.* New York: Academic Press Inc.

Adler, H. (2002). *Handbook of NLP: A manual for professional communicators.* Portland: Scitech Book News.

Bandura, A. (1997). Self-efficacy: The exercise of control. New York: Freeman.

Barzini, L. (1993). *The Europeans.* New York: Simon & Schuster.

Battino, Dr. Rubin, (2000). Guided imagery & other approaches to healing, NY: Crown House

Battino, R. (2007). Expectation: Principles and practice of very brief therapy. *Contemporary Hypnosis, 24(1), 19-29.*

Baumgartner, E., Finckh, A., Cedraschi, C., & Vischer, T. L. (2002, July). A six year prospective study of a cohort of patients with fibromyalgia. *Annals Rheumatology, 61(7), 644-645.*

Bennett, R. M., & Jacobsen, S. (1994). Muscle function and origin of pain in fibromyalgia. Baillieres Best Practical Clinical Rheumatology, 8(4), 721-746.

Bennett, R. M. (1995). Fibromyalgia: The commonest cause of widespread pain. *Frontiers, 21(6), 269-275.*

Bensen, H., & Stuart, E. (1993). The wellness book: A comprehensive guide to maintaining health and treating stress-related illness. New York: Fireside.

Benson, H. (1997). Timeless healing: The power and biology of belief. New York:Simon & Schuster.

Benson, H., Corliss, J., & Cowley, G. (2004, September). Brain check. *Newsweek,* 144, 44-47.

Benson, H., & Proctor, W. (2003). Triggers for a Happier Life. *Saturday Evening Post, 275(4), 38-39.*

Braden, G. (2011). The spontaneous healing of belief. Hay House, Inc. Carlsbad, CA. p. 56

Brody, H. (2000). The placebo response: How you can release the body's inner pharmacy for better health. New York: Cliff Street Books.

Brody, H. (2000, July). The placebo response: Recent research and implications *for family medicine. The Journal of Family Practice, 49, 65-66.*

Brown, W. A. (1998). The placebo effect: Should doctors be prescribing sugar pills? *Scientific American, 278(1), 90-95.*

Bunce, S. C., Larsen, R. J., & Peterson, C. (1995). Life after trauma: Personality and daily life experience of traumatized people. *Journal of Personality, 63, 165-188.*

Byrne, M. (2001, April). Understanding life experiences through a Phenomenological approach to research. Association of PeriOperative Regiesterd Nurses Journal, *73(4), 830.*

Caudill, M., Schnable, R., Zuttermeister, P. C., Benson, H., & Friedman, R. (1991). Decreased clinic utilization by chronic pain patients: Response to behavioral *medicine intervention. Clinical Journal of Pain, 7, 305-10.*

Chakrabarty, Sangita, Zoorob, & Roger. (2007). Fibromyalgia. *American Academy of Family Physicians, 76, 247-248.*

Chan, E. (2008 June). Quality of efficacy research in complementary and alternative *medicine. Journal of the American Medical Association, 299, 2685-2686.*

Copen, L. (2002, Sept/Oct). But you look so good! *Indian Life and Style Magazine, 23(2), 7.*

Cornell, A. W. (1996). *The power of focusing.* Oakland, CA: New Harbinger.

Creswell, J. W. (1998). *Qualitative inquiry and research design: Choosing among five traditions.* Thousand Oaks, CA: Sage.

Crum, A. & Langer, E. (2007, February). Mind-set matters: Exercise and the placebo *effect. Association for Psychological Science, 18(2),* 165.

Davis, G., & White, T. (n.d., 2006). *Goal attainment and pain management: A preliminary study with older adults.* Poster session presented at the annual meeting of the American Pain Society, Texas Woman's University, Denton, TX.

Dingley, C., & Roux, G. (2003). Inner strength in older Hispanic women with *chronic illness. Journal of Cultural Diversity, 10, 11-22.*

Dreaver, J. (1996). The ultimate cure. Llewelln Pulbications, St. Paul, MN

Emery, M. (2000). The intuitive healer: Accessing your inner physician. New York: St. Martin's Griffin.

Epstein, S. & Katz, L. (1992). Coping ability, stress, productive load, and symptoms. *Journal of Personality and Social Psychology, 62(5), 813-825.*

Evans, M., & Townsend, C. (n.d., 2006). *Pain catastrophizing: Putting a new Spin on the "fear factor" with chronic pain.* Poster session presented at the annual meeting of the American Pain Society, Mayo Clinic, Rochester, MN.

Evans, M. (2006). *Natural Healing.* Barnes & Noble Publishing, Inc. by arrangement with Anness Publishing Limited, New York

Fawzy, F. I., et al. (1993). Malignant melanoma: Effects of an early structured psychiatric intervention, coping and affective state on recurrence and survival 6 years later. Archives of General Psychiatry, 50, 681-89.

Gendlin, E. T. (1999). Focusing oriented psychotherapy: A manual of the Experiential method. New York: Guiford.

Gerwin, R. D. (1995). A study of 96 subjects examined both for fibromyalgia and myofascial pain. Journal of Musculoskelital Pain, 3(Suppl 1), 121

Gerwin, R. D. (1999). Differential diagnosis of myofascial pain syndrome and *fibromyalgia. Journal of Musculoskelital Pain, 7(1-2), 209-215.*

Gesell, I. (2007). Am I talking to me? The power of internal dialogue to help or *hinder our success. Journal for Quality and Participation, 30(2), 20-21.*

Glaser, R., & Kiecolt-Glaser, J. (2005, March). Stress-induced immune dysfunction:*Implications for health. Nature Reviews/Immunology, 5, 243.*

Goldberg, G. M., Kerns, R. D., & Rosenberg, R. (1993). Pain-relevant support as a buffer from depression among chronic pain patients low in instrumental *activity. Clinical Journal of Pain, 9(1), 34-40.*

Grayson, S. (1997). Spiritual healing: A simple guide for the healing of body, mind *and Spirit.* New York: Simon & Schuster.

Grayson, S. (1997). Spiritual healing: a guide for the healing of body, mind and spirit. Simon & Schuster, NY pp.63-64

Greenberg, G. (2003). Is it prozac? Or placebo? *Mother Jones,* 76-81.

Hamilton, N., Affleck, G., Tennen, H.,

Karlson, C., Luxton, D., Preacher, K., & Templin, J. (2008). Fibromyalgia: The role of sleep in affect and in negative event reactivity and recovery. *Health Psychology, 127*(4).

Harmon, W. W. (1991). On the shape of a new science. *International Center for Integrative Studies,* 21(1), 50-55.

Harvard Women's Health Watch (January, 2004). *The best way to treat fibromyalgia,. 4-5.*

Hay, L. (2000). *You can heal your life. Carlsbad, Ca:* Hay House, Inc.

Hekmat, H., Staats, P., & Staats, A. (n.d., 2006). *Do spiritual fantasies facilitate coping with acute pain?* Poster session presented at the annual meeting of the American Pain Society, University of Hawaii, Honolulu, HI.

Hellman, C. J., Budd, M., Borysenko, J., McClelland, D. C., & Hendricks, M. (2007). Focusing-oriented experiential psychotherapy: How to do it. *American Journal of Psychotherapy, 61(3), 271.*

Hinterkopf, E. (1998). Integrating spirituality in counseling: A manual for using the experiential focusing method. Alexandria, VA: American Counseling Association.

Holdcraft, L. C., Asefi, N., & Buchwalk, D. (2003, August). Complementary and alternative medicine in fibromyalgia and related symptoms. *Best Practical Research of Clinical Rheumatology, 17(4), 667-683.*

Hoffman, G. A., Harrington, A., & Fields, H. L. (2005). Pain and the placebo: What *we have learned. Perspectives in Biology and Medicine, 48(2), 262.*

Hofling, C. K. (1955, June). The place of placebos in medical practice. *General Practice, 11(6), 103-107.*

Iberg, J. (1991). Focusing. In Corsini R. (Ed.), *Handbook of Innovative Psychotherapy*. New York: Wiley Publishing.

Imamura, S. T., Lin, T.Y., Yriyrits, M. J., Fischer, S. S., Azze, R. J., & Rosgano, L.A., et al. (1997). The importance of myofascial pain syndrome in reflex *sympathetic* dystrophy. Physicians Medical Rehabilitation Clinics of North America, 8(1), 207-211.

Ingerman, S. (1991). Soul retrieval: Mending the fragmented self. San Francisco, CA: Harper Collins.

Inui, T. S. (1994, December). The Economist Magazine, 89-90.

Jahnke, R. (1999). *The healer within: Using traditional Chinese techniques to release* your body's own medicine. New York: Harper Collins.

Jensen, M., & Patterson, D. (2007). Hypnotherapy for the management of chronic pain. International Journal of Clinical and Experimental Hypnosis, 55(3).

Jones, Maureen M. (2010) What sparks disease? Association for Humanistic Psychology - Perspective. June/July, 15-17.

Juhan, D. (1987). *Job's body: A handbook for bodywork*. Barrytown, NY: Station Hill Press, Inc.

Kabat-Zinn, J. (2005). Coming to our senses. Healing ourselves and the world through mindfulness. London: Piatkus

Keen, E. A. (1975). Doing psychology phenomenologically: Methodological considerations. Unpublished manuscript, 2nd draft, Bucknell University, Lewisburg, PA.

King, S.J., Wessel, J., Bhambhami, Y., Sholter, D., & Maksymowych,W. (2002). Predictors of success of intervention programs for persons with fibromyalgia – *part 2. NeuroRehabilitation, 17(1). 41-48.*

Klagsbrun, J. (2001). A focusing approach to life-changing Illness (Video tape). Canada: Nada Lou Productions.

Klagsbrun, J. (2001, March). Listening and focusing: Holistic health care tools for *nurses. Holistic Nursing Care, 36(1).*

Kopp, M. S., & Rethelyi, J. (2004). Where psychology meets physiology: Chronic stress and premature mortality – the central-eastern European health paradox. *Brain Research Bulletin, 62, 351-367.*

Kratz, A., Davis, M., & Zautra, A. (2007). Pain acceptance moderates the relation between pain and negative affect in female osteoarthritis and fibromyalgia *patients. Annals Behavior Medicine, 33(3), 291-301.*

Langer, E. J. (1990). *Mindfulness. R*eading, M: Addison-Wesley Publishing Company.

Leijssen, M. (2007). Making space for the inner guide. *American Journal of Psychotherapy, 61(3).*

Lemp, H., Hatch, S., Carville, S., & Choy, E. (2009). Patients Experiences of living with and receiving treatment for fibromyalgia syndrome: A qualitative study. *Biomedcentral, 10(124).*

Levine, J., Gordon, N., & Fields, H. (1978). The mechanism of placebo analgesia. *The Lancet, 2, 654-657.*

Limer, K., Nicholl, B., Thomson, W., & McBeth, J. (2007). Exploring the genetic susceptibility of chronic widespread pain: The tender points in genetic *association studies. Rheumatology, 47, 572-577.*

Lipton, B. (2005). The biology of belief: Unleashing the power of consciousness matter and miracles. Santa Rosa, Ca: Mountain of Love/Elite books.

Long, T. (2004). The fibromyalgia dilemma. *Journal of Controversial Medical* Claims, 11(1), 2

McCracken, l., Gauntlett-Gilbert, J., & Vowles, K. (n.d., 2007). Mindfulness, chronic pain-related suffering, and disability: A contextual cognitive-behavioral *analysis*. Poster presented at the annual meeting of the Pain Management Unit, Royal National Hospital for Rheumatic Diseases and University of Bath. Bath, UK.

McDermott, I., & O'Connor, J. (1996). *NLP and health*. San Francisco, CA: Harper Collins Publishers.

McDermott, I., & Jago, W. (2002, September). *Brief NLP therapy*. Portland: Scitech Book News, 26(3).

McEwen, B., & Lasley, E. N (2002). The end of stress as we know it. *Washington*, DC: National Academies Press.

McEwen, B. S., & Seeman, T. (1999). Protective and damaging effects of mediators of stress: Elaborating and testing the concepts of allostasis and allostatic load. *Annals of the New York Academy of Sciences, 896, 30-47.*

McGraw, P. (2001). Self Matters: Creating your life from the inside out. New York:Simon & Schuster.

McNicol, T. (1996), April). The new faith in medicine. USA Weekend, 5-7.

Mehl-Madrona, L. (2003). Coyote Medicine: What traditional Native Americans can teach us about healing. Paper presented at NICABM Conference, Hilton Head, NC.

Mehl-Madrona, L. (2003). Healing as an adventure. *Advances in Mind-body Medicine, 19(2), 19.*

Meili, T., & Kabat-Zinn, J. (2004). The power of the human heart: A story of trauma and recovery and its implications for rehabilitation and healing. *Journal of Phenomenological Psychology, 20(1), 6-16.*

Menzies, V., Gill Taylor, A., & Bourguignon, C. (2006). Effects of guided imagery on outcomes of pain, functional status, and self-efficacy in persons diagnosed *with Fibromyalgia. The Journal of Alternative and Complementary Medicine, 12(1), 23–30.*

Metal'nikov, S. (1934). Role de systeme nerveux et des facteurs biologiques et *psychiques dans l'immunite. [The role of the nervous system and biological and physiological factors for immunity]. Paris: Masson.*

Miller, W. R. (1997). Spiritual aspects of addictions treatment and research. M*ind/Body Medicine, 2(1), 37-43.*

Milstein, J. (2008, July). Introducing spirituality in medical care, transition from hopelessness to wholeness. Journal of the American Medical Association, *2440-2441.*

Molton, I., Graham, C., Stoelb, B., & Jensen, M. (2007, October). Current Psychological approaches to the management of chronic pain. *Current Opinion in Anaesthesiology, 20(5), 485-489.*

Morone, N., Lynch, C., Greco, C., Tindle, H., & Weiner, D. (2008, September). I felt like a new person: The effects of mindfulness meditation on older adults with chronic pain. Journal of Pain, 841(8).

Morris, V., S. Cruwys, & B. Kidd. (1998). Increased capsaicin-induced secondary hyperalgesia as a marker of abnormal sensory activity in patients with Fibromyalgia. Neuroscience Letters, 260(3), 205-7.

Moustakas, C. (1994). Phenomenological research methods. Thousand Oaks, CA:Sage Publications.

Munce, S., & Stewart, D. (2007). Gender differences in depression and chronic pain conditions in a national epidemiologic survey. The Academy of Psychosomatic Medicine, 48, 394-300.

Myss, C. (1997). Why people don't heal and how they can. New York: Three Rivers Press.

National Institute of Arthritis and Musculoskeletal and Skin Diseases. (2004, June). Questions and answers about fibromyalgia. *National Institute of Health, 04-5326, 1-4.*

Naparstek, Belleruth (1994) Staying well with guided imagery. NY: Warner Books

Newman, A. L., & Peterson, C. (1996). Anger of women incest survivors. *Sex roles, 34, 463-474.*

Nijs, L., & Van Houdenhove, B. (2008). From acute musculoskeletal pain to chronic widespread pain and fibromyalgia: Application of pain neurophysiology in *manual therapy practice. Manual Therapy, 03, 1-10.*

Noller, V., & Sprott, H. (2003, August). Prospective epidemiological observations on the course of the disease in fibromyalgia patients. *Journal of Negative Results Biomedicine, 2(1), 4.*

Nunley, A. (1999). *Inner counselor.* NewYork: Sterling House.

Park, L. C., & Covi, L. (1965). Nonblind placebo trial. *Archives of General Psychiatry, 12, 336-345.*

Pelletier, K. (1994). *Sound mind, sound body.* New York: Simon & Schuster.

Pelletier, K. (2000). The best alternative medicine: What works? What does not? New York: Simon & Schuster.

Pelletier, K. (2002). Mind as healer, mind as slayer: Mindbody medicine comes of *age. Advances in Mind Body Medicine, 18(1), 14-15.*

Pert, C. (1997). *Molecules of emotion.* New York: Scribner.

Pert, C. (2002). The wisdom of the receptors: Neuropeptides, the emotions and *bodymind. Advances in Medicine, 18(1), 30-35.*

Roberts, T. B. (2000, September). Somatosensory-hypnotherapy: Integrating Mindbody and hypnotherapeutic approaches to facilitate symptom release. *Australian Journal of clinical Hypnotherapy and Hypnosis.*

Rooks, D. (2007). Fibromyalgia treatment update. *Current Opinion in Rheumatology, 19, 111-117.*

Rooks, D., Gautam, S., Romeling, M., Cross, M., Stratigakis, D., Evans, B.,Goldenberg, D., Iversen, M., & Katz, J. (2007). Group exercise, education, and combination self-management in women with fibromyalgia. *Archives Internal medicine, 167(20), 2192-2200.*

Rubenfeld, I. (1997, September). An interview with Ilana Rubenfeld. *Family Therapy Networker.*

Russell, I. J. (1999). Is fibromyalgia a distinct clinical entity? The clinical investigator's evidence. Baillieres Best Practical Research Clinical Rheumatology, 13(3), 445

Salkeld, E. (2008, January). Integrative medicine and clinical practice: Diagnosis *and treatment strategies. Complementary Health Practice Revie, 13(1), 21.*

Santorelli, S. (1992). Heal thyself: Lessons on mindfulness in medicine. New York: Bell Tower.

Scascighini, L., Toma, V., Dober-Spielmann, S., & Sprott, H. (2008). Multidisciplinary treatment for chronic pain: A systematic review of interventions and outcomes. *Rheumatology, 47(5), 670-678.*

Segerstrom, S. C., & Miller, G. E. (2004). Psychological stress and the human immune system: A meta-analytic study of 30 years of inquiry. *Psychological Bulletin, 130(4), 601-630.*

Sharoff, L. (2008). Exploring nurses' perceived benefits of utilizing holistic Modalities for self and clients. *Holistic Nursing Practice, 22(1), 15-24.*

Sherman, C. (2007, April). Fibromyalgia enters the mainstream after two decades on the fringes. *Cortland Forum, 20(8), 72.*

Shure, N. (1965). The placebo effect in allergy. *Annals of Allergy, 23,* 368-376.

Siegel, B. (1996). *Love, medicine and miracles.* New York: Harper Collins.

Siegel, B. (2002, May). *Whole person care.* Presented at the ECaP Professional Training Program. Pittsburgh, PA.

Siegel, B. (2003). Healing our lives. *Advances in Mind-Body Medicine,* 19(2), 13-14.

Simons, D. G., J. G. Travell, & L. S. Simons. (1999). *Travell and Simons' myofascial pain and dysfunction.* The Trigger Point Manual, (2nd Ed.). Baltimore: Williams and Wilkins.

Sivik, T. (2000, July/August). Psychosomatic medicine: Why fix it if it ain't broken? *Psychotherapy and Psychosomatics.*

Sivik, T. (2005). Psychosomatic integrative treatment and rehabilitation. *Advances in Medicine, 21,* 55-57.

Sobel, D. (1995). All in your head. Mental Medicine, update 3.

Sobel, D. (2000). Mind matters, money matters: The cost-effectiveness of mind/body *medicine. Journal of the American Medical Association, 284(1705), 395-396.*

Solomon, G. F. (1981). *Psychoneuroimmunology.* New York: Academic Press.

Spradley, J. (1980). *Participant observation.* New York: Holt, Rinehart & Winston.

Spiegel, D. (2008, May). What is the placebo worth? *British Medical Journal, 335(7651), 967.*

Stacks, D. W., & Andersen, P.A (1989). The modular mind: Implications for *intrapersonal communication. The Southern Communication Journal, 54,*273-293.

Starlanyl, D. (1998). *The fibromyalgia advocate.* Oakland, CA: New Harbinger Publications.

Starlanyl, D., & Copeland, M. E. (2000). *Fibromyalgia & chronic myofascial pain.* Oakland, CA: New Harbinger Publications.

Stelter, R. (2000). The transformation of body experience into language. *Journal of Phenomenological Psychology, 31(1), 63.*

Sullivan, L. W. (1991). Partners in prevention: A mobilization plan for implementing healthy people 2000. *American Journal of Health Promotion, 5(4), 291-297.*

Talbot, S. (2007) T*he Cortisol Connection: Why Stress Makes You Fat and Ruins Your Health.* Hunter House Inc.Publishers.

Targ, E. (2000, December). *Spirituality and healing: Evidence and practical applications.* Paper presented at the NICABM Conference, Hilton Head, SC.

Tausk, F., Elenkov, I., & Moynihan, J. (2008). Psychoneuroimmunology. Dermatologic Therapy, 21, 22-31.

Taylor, E. (1997). *A psychology of spiritual healing.* West Chester, PA: Chrysalis Books.

Thorson, K. (1999). Is fibromyalgia a distinct clinical entity? The patient's evidence. *Baillieres Best Practical Research Clinical Rheumatology, 13(3), 463-467.*

Treadwell, Kimberli R. H., & Kendall, Phillip C. (1996). Self-talk in youth with anxiety disorders: States of mind, content specificity, and treatment outcome. J*ournal of Consulting and Clinical Psychology, 64(5), 941-949.*

Turk, D., Swanson, K., & Tunks, E. (2008, April). Psychological approaches in the treatment of chronic pain patients – when pills, scalpels, and needles are not enough. *The Canadian Journal of Psychiatry, 53(4), 213-223.*

Vincent, D. (1994, December). Why doctors? *The Economist Magazine,* 89-90.

Vowles, K., MacLaren, J., & Gross, R. (2006). *Continued depressive symptoms as a risk of Decrease treatment effect following interdisciplinary treatment. Paper* presented at American Pain Society, 2006 Annual Meeting.

Walter, J., & Bayat, A. (2003, May). Neurolinguistic programming: Verbal Communication. Student British Medical Journal, 163.

Walter, J., & Bayat, A. (2003, July). Neurolinguistic programming: The keys to success. *Student British Medical Journal, 252-253.*

Warter, C. (December, 2000). *Spiritual applications of a clinical practice.* Presented at the NICABM Conference, Hilton Head, SC.

Wisneski, L. (1997). A unified energy field theory of physiology and healing. *Stress Medicine, 13, 259-265.*

Wisneski, L. (1999, October). Psychoneuroimmunology: The scientific basis of holistic medicine. *The Integrative Medicine Consult, 1(15), 135.*

Wittrup, I. H., Wiik, A., & Danneskild-Samsoe, B. (1999). Antibody profile in patients with fibromyalgia compared to healthy controls. *Journal of Musculoskel* Pain, 7(1-2), 273-277.

Wolfe, F., Anderson, J., Harkness, D., Bennett, R. M., Caro, X. J., Goldenberg, D., L., Russell, I. J., & Yunus, M. B. (1997). Health status and disease severity of fibromyalgia: Results of a six-center longitudinal study. *Arthritis Rheumatism, 40(9), 1571-1579.*

Zautra, A., Parrish, B., Puymbroeck, C., Tennen, H., Davis, M., Reich, J., & Irwin, M. (2007, June). Depression history, stress, and pain in rheumatoid arthritis patients. *Journal of Behavioral Medicine, 30(3), 18*

Zautra, A. (2008, July). Strengthening resilience capacity might light the way to a brighter future for patients with fibromyalgia. *Nature Clinical Practice,* 1-2.

Ziemssen, T., & Kern, S. (2007). Pychoneuroimmunology – Cross-talk between the immune and nervous systems. *Journal of Neurology, 254*(11), 8-11.

www.ingramcontent.com/pod-product-compliance
Lightning Source LLC
Chambersburg PA
CBHW051639170526
45167CB00001B/255